Dear Future Exam Success Story

First of all, **THANK YOU** for purchasing Mometrix study materials!

Second, congratulations! You are one of the few determined test-takers who are committed to doing whatever it takes to excel on your exam. **You have come to the right place.** We developed these practice tests with one goal in mind: to deliver you the best possible approximation of the questions you will see on test day.

Standardized testing is one of the biggest obstacles on your road to success, which only increases the importance of doing well in the high-pressure, high-stakes environment of test day. Your results on this test could have a significant impact on your future, and these practice tests will give you the repetitions you need to build your familiarity and confidence with the test content and format to help you achieve your full potential on test day.

Your success is our success

We would love to hear from you! If you would like to share the story of your exam success or if you have any questions or comments in regard to our products, please contact us at **800-673-8175** or **support@mometrix.com**.

Thanks again for your business and we wish you continued success!

Sincerely,
The Mometrix Test Preparation Team

AF834554

Written and edited by the Mometrix Exam Secrets Test Prep Team
Printed in the United States of America

CHES

Exam

Practice Questions

Mometrix
TEST PREPARATION

TABLE OF CONTENTS

Practice Test #1

1. If advising members of the general public about the most valid online source for health information, the health education specialist should advise them to look for URLs that end with:

a. .org
b. .com
c. .gov
d. .edu

2. A client enrolled in a program to reduce obesity has repeatedly failed to stay on a diet and exercise program and has not lost weight. Because of the lack of weight loss, the client has concluded that the program is ineffective. Which communication theory does this exemplify?

a. cognitive dissonance
b. attribution theory
c. contextual design
d. gatekeeping theory

3. If a health education specialist working in the public health field wants to become active in a professional organization, which of the following might best meet the health education specialist's needs?

a. ASHA
b. ASPPH
c. SOPHE
d. DHPE

4. If the health education specialist is interested in using an asset-based community development strategy to implement a program, the first step is to map:

a. personal capacities and assets.
b. capacities and assets of the political resources.
c. capacities and assets needed for successful implementation.
d. capacities and assets of individuals, organizations, and institutions.

5. In order to be effective, implementation of a program of blood pressure screening and treatment should include:

a. free medications.
b. lifestyle counseling.
c. free blood pressure monitoring devices.
d. behavioral therapy.

6. The best preparation for total implementation of a program is usually:

a. written program guide.
b. targeted training.
c. pilot testing.
d. adequate resources.

7. Which Boolean operator would be used to search for synonymous terms/concepts?

a. OR
b. AND
c. NOT
d. NEAR

8. Which of the following is an example of an interpersonal channel of communication?

a. workplace campaigns
b. newsletters
c. town hall meetings
d. hotline counseling

9. If the health education specialist is utilizing the Critical Path Method (CPM) work plan when planning a project, which step must be completed first?

a. Identify resources.
b. Identify costs.
c. Identify activities.
d. Identify timeline.

10. Which government agency can provide the most extensive information about diabetes mellitus?

a. NIDDK
b. CDC
c. AHRQ
d. NIMH

Questions 11 and 12 refer to the following information:

Graph 1

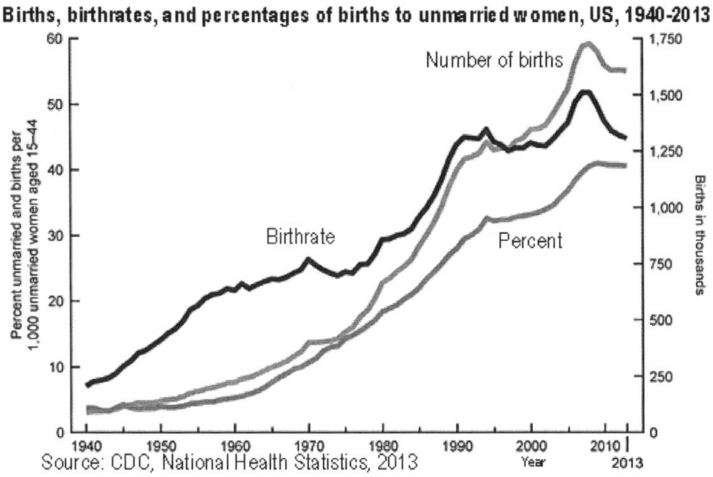

11. The health education specialist is planning an education program for new mothers and is reviewing the trends in births to unmarried women. Based on Graph 1, since 2005 the birthrate among unmarried women ages 15-44 in the United States has:

a. increased.
b. decreased.
c. stabilized.
d. fluctuated up and down.

12. According to Graph 1, the decade in which the number of births to unmarried women increased the most is:

a. 1950-1960.
b. 1960-1970.
c. 1970-1980.
d. 1980-1990.

13. Under the HIPAA privacy rule, health information may be used for research purposes without patient authorization if it is:

a. de-identified.
b. individually identifiable.
c. necessary for analysis.
d. in the public good.

14. All of the following are likely to hinder the acquisition of skills except:

a. lack of motivation.
b. moderate anxiety.
c. complex task.
d. environmental noise.

15. The most effective method of teaching participants in a program the technical skills needed to use electronic equipment is:

a. trial and error.
b. hands-on practice.
c. video guide.
d. written manual.

16. When completing a review of literature as part of quantitative research, the review of literature should be carried out:

a. after data are collected.
b. at the end of the research process.
c. at the beginning of the research process.
d. whenever convenient for the researchers.

17. When carrying out a critical appraisal of a quantitative study, the first step in determining the validity of a quantitative study is:

a. evaluation.
b. analysis.
c. comparison.
d. comprehension.

18. When the health education specialist is training personnel to assist with data collection, which of the following is most critical?

a. consistency
b. timeframe
c. costs
d. attitude

19. The four primary tasks in data collection are (1) selecting subjects, (2) collecting data systematically, (3) maintaining research controls, and (4):

a. evaluating variables.
b. solving problems.
c. utilizing resources.
d. maintaining consistency.

20. At what point in an advocacy program should advocacy evaluation be considered?

a. before implementation of the program
b. periodically during implementation
c. during the planning stages
d. after the program has concluded or after a specified period of time

Questions 21-23 refer to the following information:

Scenario A

Because of the high rate of obesity, hypertension, and diabetes mellitus, type 2, among Mexican immigrant families, the health education specialist is planning a multi-level program that will include vouchers to a free health clinic for health checkups and follow-up, a farmer's market each Sunday at one of the major churches serving the community to encourage the use of fresh fruits and vegetables, removal of sugar-laden drinks from vending machines at schools and recreation centers, renovation of a local park to encourage activity, and community workshops to educate people about diet and exercise.

21. The health education specialist has not worked with a Mexican immigrant population before. When tasked with developing an educational program for an immigrant group with whom the health education specialist is not familiar, before beginning course development, the best approach is to:

a. read about the target population.
b. apply general educational principles.
c. interview members of the target population.
d. ask other health education specialists for advice.

22. The health education specialist conducts observations, interviews, and surveys to better understand the community's needs. When families of immigrants from Mexico are asked to participate in interviews and other activities about the needs of immigrants, the decision to participate is likely to be made by the:

a. mother.
b. father.
c. extended family member.
d. priest/minister.

23. What type of strategy is utilized when replacing sugar-laden drinks in vending machines in schools and recreation centers with juice or sugar-free drinks?

a. community mobilization
b. health engineering
c. enforcement
d. community service

24. If a potential research subject is led to believe that the individual's medical care will be adversely affected if the individual does not participate in a research project, this is an example of:

a. deception.
b. confusion.
c. coercion.
d. negligence.

25. When the health education specialist is collecting data in the community about substance abuse and comparing it to national data, a good secondary source of data is:

a. SAMHSA.
b. CDC.
c. CMS.
d. FDA.

26. If a needs assessment includes the observation that local health clinics are serving large numbers of pregnant adolescents, the type of need this represents is:

a. normative.
b. perceived.
c. expressed.
d. comparative.

27. Which of the following is a social determinant that can impact health?

a. increased sales tax on alcoholic beverages
b. toxic exposures
c. poor street lighting
d. increased exposure to mass media

28. Which of the following factors is likely to have the least influence on health behaviors?

a. age
b. place of residence
c. socioeconomic status
d. social support network

29. Which of the following emerging trends may have the most influence on health?

a. legalization of marijuana
b. decriminalization of drug offenses
c. use of e-cigarettes
d. increased use of social media

30. Which of the following resources for assessment generally has the least financial and time costs?

a. surveys (paper)
b. interviews
c. surveys (online)
d. secondary data

31. When developing a vision statement, the vision should focus on:

a. past achievements.
b. current status.
c. future goals.
d. financial stability.

32. When preparing an audiovisual presentation, which type of display is most appropriate for continuous data?

a. histogram
b. line graph
c. bar chart
d. pie chart

33. Emotional readiness to learn is most affected by:

a. past coping mechanisms.
b. current knowledge base.
c. gender.
d. motivation.

34. The health education specialist regularly communicates directions and status updates to staff members regarding a program being implemented in the form of read-only e-mails. The primary problem with this form of communication is that it:

a. is uninteresting.
b. has limited audience reach.
c. is one-way.
d. may be overlooked.

35. If the health education specialist wants to begin an advocacy campaign to increase the number of shelters for the homeless in order to reduce illness and injury among the homeless population, the first step is to:

a. notify the media.
b. gather allies and supporters.
c. call for a rally.
d. inundate politicians with telephone calls.

36. If using the 4-part method of writing objectives, which component is inadequate in this objective?

"Following a class on HIV prevention, the participants will be able to describe transmission."

a. condition/testing situation
b. learner
c. performance
d. criterion for mastery

37. If a needs assessment indicates a need for a program within the community to combat childhood obesity, the resource that is probably most critical is:

a. political.
b. social.
c. financial.
d. environmental.

38. When prioritizing needs for health education, the first step is to:

a. identify criteria.
b. identify interventions.
c. determine voting procedures.
d. assess costs.

39. Which of the following is an appropriate goal statement?

a. Provide classes in smoking cessation to adolescents.
b. Provide emergency shelter for the homeless.
c. Lower the cost of health care through prevention strategies.
d. Teach parents strategies to prevent childhood obesity.

Questions 40 and 41 refer to the following information:

Graph 2

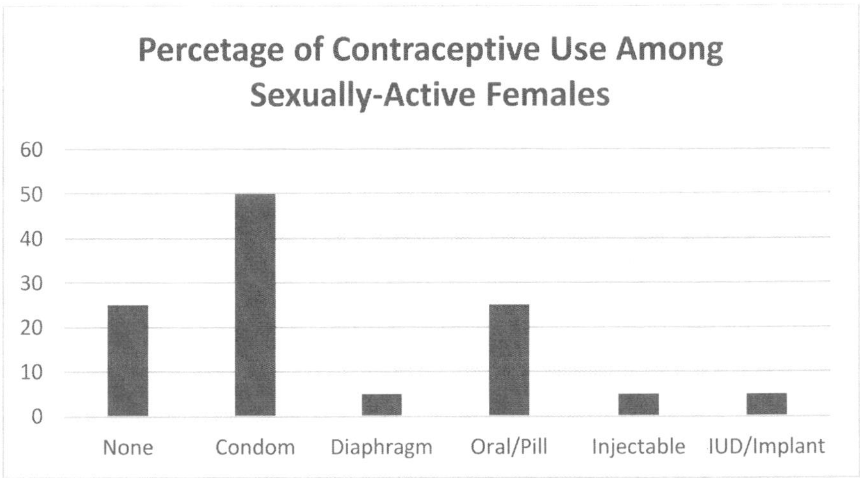

40. In order to assess the need for an educational program to reduce sexually transmitted diseases (STDs) at a university, the health education specialist conducted a survey to determine the types of contraception and protection consistently used by female students. Based on the data illustrated in Graph 2, approximately what percentage of sexually active females uses both a condom and another form of birth control?

a. 15%
b. 25%
c. 55%
d. 75%

41. Using the data illustrated in Graph 2, the health education specialist develops an education plan about safe sex. Which group of students should be considered as the target audience?

a. all students
b. female students only
c. male students only
d. students not using condoms

42. Which of the following is an example of a demographic factor that may be considered when identifying a priority population?

a. school currently attending
b. community of residence
c. agency/organization
d. level of education

43. As a member of an advocacy group who is trying to develop a halfway house for substance abusers in a neighborhood, the health education specialist is confronted by people who are adamantly opposed to the project. The best initial response is to:

a. disregard those who are opposed.
b. try to change the minds of those opposed.
c. determine the reason for the opposition.
d. recruit advocates in order to outnumber those in opposition.

44. When eliciting input about a health education plan for a priority population, input that is most critical usually comes from the:

a. social services.
b. priority population.
c. healthcare providers.
d. political representatives.

45. When a number of different advocacy groups are all focused on one goal or issue, such as improving women's health, this is an example of a:

a. community of ideas.
b. community of memory.
c. community of crisis.
d. community of circumstance.

46. When designing interventions to reduce risk-taking behavior in a population, the ethical principle that is applied when the health education specialist assures participants that use of illicit drugs will not be reported to the police is:

a. veracity.
b. beneficence.
c. confidentiality.
d. non-malfeasance.

47. When planning an outreach program for the homeless community, the best place to provide information about the program to people who are homeless and may benefit is likely:

a. in shelters and soup kitchens.
b. on the street.
c. in churches.
d. at community centers.

48. The best way for the health education specialist to ensure a commitment from individuals to participate in an educational program is to:

a. ask people if they are committed.
b. assist people to pre-register.
c. send out literature asking for telephone registration.
d. charge a fee.

49. When searching for a facility in which to hold classes for a priority population, the health education specialist's first consideration should be:

a. size of room.
b. cost for space.
c. lighting.
d. ADA compliance.

50. If the goal is to encourage active participation among all class members, the best seating arrangement for a group of 10 participants is:

a. in standard rows.
b. around tables
c. in a circle.
d. wherever participants feel comfortable.

51. Which of the following would be an activity in media advocacy?

a. Taking part in lobbying activities.
b. Writing op-ed articles.
c. Speaking one-on-one to individuals.
d. Participating in conference presentations.

52. For a slide presentation (such as with PowerPoint) that is to accompany a lecture, a well-designed presentation should NOT contain:

a. complete lecture text.
b. sans serif font.
c. bulleted highlights.
d. illustrations/diagrams.

53. If the health education specialist has conducted a media campaign to increase HPV vaccinations of both boys and girls at two local clinics, the best method to evaluate the impact is to:

a. conduct a general public survey of opinions about HPV vaccinations.
b. monitor rates of HPV infections.
c. interview physicians.
d. monitor the number of vaccinations provided.

54. Determining whether an education program was worth the investment and should be continued is part of:

a. summative evaluation.
b. formative evaluation.
c. content evaluation.
d. impact evaluation.

55. During phase I of the PRECEDE-PROCEED model, the type of assessment carried out is:

a. educational/ecological.
b. epidemiological.
c. social.
d. administrative/policy.

56. If the health education specialist is involved in an advocacy group with a national focus, the best way to gain local supporters is to:

a. focus on local issues that are related.
b. focus on national needs.
c. explain how the national focus may have a local impact.
d. appeal to people's altruism.

Questions 57 and 58 refer to the following information:

Scenario B

Two nonprofit agencies have formed a partnership and are applying for a joint federal grant but must negotiate to determine how the grant money will be divided between the agencies. The leaders from both agencies meet and attempt to determine how best to meet the financial needs of both agencies.

57. This negotiation style is:

a. compromising.
b. accommodative.
c. competitive.
d. collaborative.

58. When two agencies form a partnership, what type of resource does the partnership itself represent?

a. intellectual
b. financial
c. physical
d. human

59. The health education specialist is assessing the types of problems that developed in the implementation of a program and whether the resources and training were adequate to achieve the desired results. This is an example of:

a. outcomes evaluation.
b. formative evaluation.
c. process evaluation.
d. impact evaluation.

60. When planning learning assignments, the health education specialist should realize that the least retention is likely to occur with:

a. practicing/restating.
b. reading.
c. listening.
d. seeing.

61. If giving a presentation to a community group about the results of a health prevention strategy, the best method to convey the statistical changes is likely:

a. line chart.
b. table.
c. narrative.
d. raw data.

62. When the health education specialist is evaluating instructional methods, the most important issue is whether the method:

a. addresses different learning styles.
b. is easily accessible by learner.
c. has costs involved.
d. helps learners achieve goals and objectives.

63. After a series of deaths from fires and carbon monoxide poisonings in an immigrant community, a preventive program to install free smoke and carbon monoxide alarms is unsuccessful when community members refuse to allow admission into their homes. The best solution is to:

a. discontinue the program.
b. offer free alarms and instructions at community gathering places.
c. advertise availability of free alarms at fire departments.
d. have police accompany volunteers who are installing alarms.

64. A typical logic model contains (1) inputs, (2) activities, (3) outputs, and (4):

a. outcomes/impacts.
b. resources.
c. literature review.
d. statistics.

65. Pilot studies are used for all of the following reasons except to:

a. determine feasibility.
b. guide modifications.
c. assess long-term outcomes.
d. examine reliability, validity, and usability.

66. Which of the following factors is most likely to foster implementation of an educational program?

a. media support
b. community support
c. marketing plan
d. legislative guidelines

67. The health education specialist observes a staff member involved in a health program for adolescents being physically abusive to a participant. Who among the others who were present is a mandated reporter and must contact the legal authorities?

a. social worker
b. program participant
c. volunteer
d. contract housekeeping staff

68. Skill inoculation refers to:

a. one-on-one instruction.
b. utilization of different learning styles.
c. repeated practice of tasks.
d. repeated observations of tasks.

69. If developing a substance abuse program for homeless veterans in a residential community where residents have resisted such programs in the past, the health education specialist should:

a. consult an attorney regarding legal liability.
b. avoid notifying the residents.
c. notify the residents after the program is implemented.
d. notify the residents in advance.

70. Prior to beginning the first phase of implementation of a new program, the health education specialist should:

a. survey all stakeholders.
b. notify the media.
c. review the program budget.
d. ensure sustainability.

71. When recruiting individuals needed for implementation of an education plan, the health education specialist should first:

a. write a series of interview questions.
b. develop a job description.
c. determine the salary for paid positions.
d. determine the desired personal characteristics.

72. When collecting baseline data prior to implementation of a program, the first place to begin is usually:

a. ask other professionals for information.
b. focus groups.
c. secondary data collection.
d. primary data collection.

73. The first step in securing resources to implement a plan is to identify the:

a. resources needed.
b. existing resources.
c. potential sources of resources.
d. budgetary allowance for resources.

74. If searching a database for lists of journal articles in the field of biomedics, the best resource is:

a. CINAHL.
b. ERIC.
c. HEDIR.
d. MEDLINE.

75. When conducting a survey, the type of questions that are the most difficult to quantify are:

a. true/false.
b. multiple choice.
c. open-ended.
d. rating scale.

76. When using a Program Evaluation and Review Technique (PERT) chart for time management, the three time estimates that should be included for each activity are:

a. beginning, midpoint, and ending.
b. optimistic, likely, and pessimistic.
c. starting, projected, and ending.
d. starting, expected, and overages.

77. Organizational readiness for implementation is exemplified by all of the following except:

a. commitment to change.
b. ability to bring about change.
c. positive attitudes toward change.
d. establishment of timeline for implementation.

78. If a pop-up message promoting a health program appears on an individual's computer screen based on the individual's browsing history of gyms, weight loss programs, and health-related sites, this is an example of a:

a. tailored message.
b. targeted message.
c. spam message.
d. random message.

79. If a health education program that was presented in group classes is to be updated so the material can be presented on the internet, the most cost-effective approach is generally to:

a. discard existing materials and start over.
b. purchase a commercial program.
c. assess, modify, and utilize existing materials.
d. scan materials and use without modification.

80. If utilizing the social-ecological model when developing preventive strategies, the first level focuses on the:

a. society.
b. community.
c. relationships.
d. individual.

81. A recent outbreak of severe nausea and vomiting has been traced to use of a banned pesticide, and the health education specialist must develop an educational campaign to warn the public. The first step in identifying the priority population is to:

a. study the distribution of cases and demographic information.
b. make an appeal in the print and broadcast media.
c. interview nursery owners and other places that sell plants.
d. contact individuals who have been treated.

82. If developing an educational program based on evidence-based research and using the RE-AIM method to improve generalizability and sustainability, the first issue to consider is:

a. recording data.
b. reaching the priority population.
c. ranking priorities.
d. recommending interventions.

83. When the health education specialist is choosing materials/interventions for an education program, the most important consideration is that the materials/interventions be:

a. cost-effective.
b. supported by the priority population.
c. evidence-based.
d. easy to understand and simple to use.

84. In order to adequately evaluate the outcomes of interventions, it is necessary that there be intervention:

a. retention.
b. repetition.
c. limitation.
d. fidelity.

Questions 58 refers to the following information:

Graph 3

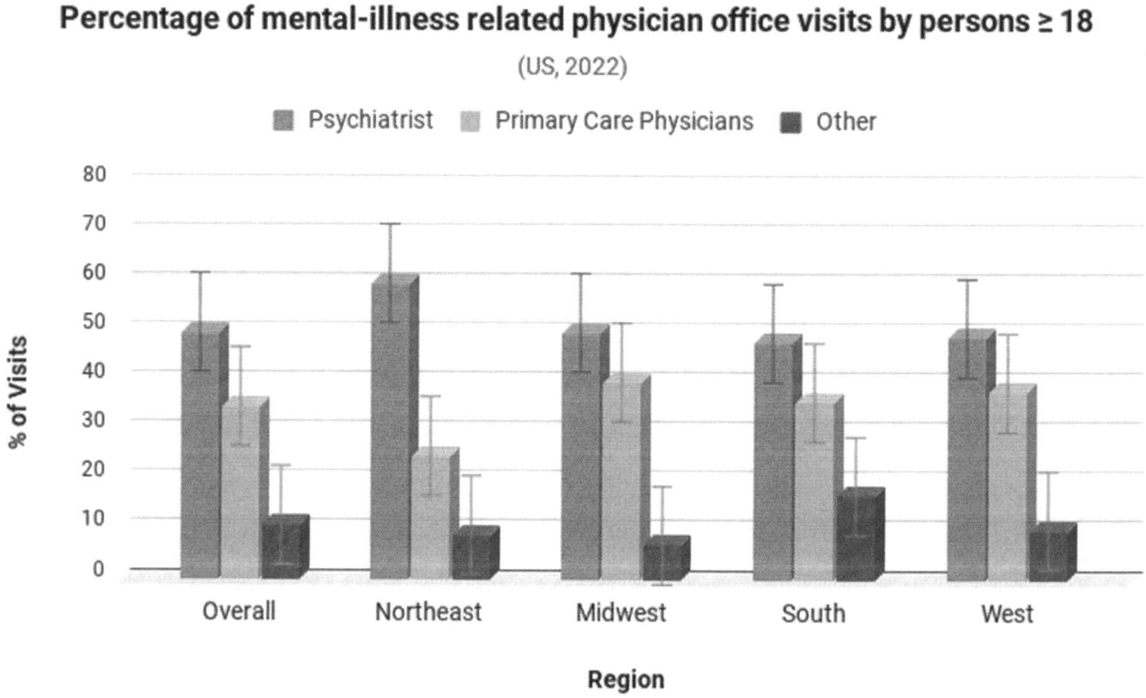

85. Based on the information in Graph 3, in which area of the country are people 18 years and older more likely to consult a psychiatrist for mental illness–related disorder than a primary care physicians or other physician?

a. Midwest
b. Northeast
c. West
d. South

86. Which of the following is an example of an impact objective?

a. By 2025, pregnancy rates of adolescents in the Sandcity community will decrease by 50%.
b. By June 2023, surveys of adolescents in the Sandcity community will indicate a 25% increase in the use of condoms.
c. By June 2023, at least 80% of adolescents who were provided literature are aware of the need to practice birth control.
d. By June 2023, the health education specialist will have conducted 6 classes regarding preventing pregnancy for adolescents at the local high schools and community center.

87. Which of the following findings represents a need for increased capacity?

a. Organization has clear measurable objectives.
b. Organization members lack understanding of organizational vision.
c. Organizational programs are clearly defined and in line with mission and vision.
d. Ongoing evaluation identifies necessary program modifications.

88. Which of the following is usually the most important aspect of a training program?

a. equipment
b. setting
c. instructor's ability
d. time of instruction

89. When developing a marketing plan aimed at a priority population, the first element to consider is:

a. priority population.
b. cost.
c. types of media.
d. time frame.

90. Which of the following is an example of material/equipment for a low-fidelity simulation to be used for educational purposes?

a. mannequin
b. blood pressure cuff
c. AED
d. printed case study

91. As part of a community education program, the health education specialist is developing a series of podcasts. What is the longest each podcast should be to retain user interest?

a. 5 minutes
b. 10 minutes
c. 30 minutes
d. 60 minutes

92. What type of decision making is the health education specialist utilizing when making decisions about how to transmit information to individuals in an education program?

a. informative
b. targeted
c. communicative
d. preventive

93. Which of the following is an example of aggregate data?

a. physician orders
b. laboratory findings
c. good practice guidelines
d. demographic information

94. Placing ads on television about a community program to reduce drinking and driving and to provide free rides to impaired individuals is an example of utilizing:

a. paid media.
b. social media.
c. earned media.
d. digital media.

95. If an educational program at an organization is to be successful, it is most important to have:

a. financial support.
b. management support.
c. audience interest.
d. space and equipment.

96. In addition to financial support, space, and curriculum, resources critical to implementation of an education plan include:

a. personnel and supplies.
b. time and motivation.
c. personnel and motivation.
d. time and supplies.

97. Two nonprofit community agencies have agreed to implement a joint project in which both will provide different but complementary services, and have agreed to create a memorandum of understanding (MOU). The first section of the MOU should contain the:

a. starting and ending dates.
b. description of the parties involved.
c. responsibilities of the parties.
d. intent of the project.

98. If the work plan and timeline show that implementation is far behind schedule and the health education specialist plans to modify the implementation plan, the health education specialist must assess the effect that modification will have on:

a. security.
b. advocacy.
c. fidelity.
d. strategy.

99. If, as part of a health-related strategy, policies are enacted to discourage alcohol/substance misuse and institute a drug-free workplace, the first step in implementation is:

a. publishing the drug-free policy.
b. educating staff about alcohol/substance misuse.
c. providing an employee assistance program (EAP).
d. ensuring privacy for those seeking treatment.

Questions 100-102 refer to the following information:

Scenario C

A health education specialist is working in an area with three large retirement communities and is planning multi-level interventions to decrease risk of disease among senior citizens and to promote healthier lifestyles.

100. Which educational strategy is likely to be most effective for a population older than 65 years?

a. health fairs
b. social networking (Instagram/Twitter)
c. role playing
d. audiovisual/print materials

101. The health intervention specialist has planned a number of interventions. Which of the following interventions is an example of an intervention at the primary level of prevention?

a. Providing staff training regarding caring for stroke patients
b. Chairing a stroke recovery support group
c. Conducting stroke-screening tests at local pharmacies, supermarkets, and recreation centers
d. Advising local supermarkets about placing of items for wheelchair access

102. The health education specialist wants to inform people in the retirement communities of classes about diet and exercise for senior citizens, but the socioeconomic status and cultural backgrounds of the priority populations at the three retirement communities are quite different. The best initial step is:

a. internet ads.
b. newspaper ads.
c. flyers.
d. focus groups.

103. If an assessment instrument yields consistent test results in different events (test-retest), then the instrument is said to have:

a. reliability.
b. readability.
c. validity.
d. predictability.

104. Informed consent for those participating in research includes all of the following except:

a. nature/purpose of the project.
b. risks associated with participation in the project.
c. penalty for stopping participation in the project.
d. benefits of participation in the project.

105. If a web-based testing instrument assessing knowledge about food and nutrition shows similar results to one-on-one testing, the web-based instrument is said to have:

a. construct validity.
b. criterion related validity.
c. face validity.
d. content validity.

106. If data collection includes four different paper surveys and data must be evaluated on an individual as well as group basis, the best method of data storage is to use:

a. different folders for each survey for each individual.
b. color-coded surveys in individual folders.
c. computer-entered data only.
d. color-coded surveys in separate group folders.

107. If using a commercial survey company to collect and manage electronic data, it is most important for the health education specialist to investigate:

a. accessibility.
b. storage capacity.
c. costs.
d. security.

108. An institutional review board (IRB) must be comprised of at least:

a. 3 members.
b. 5 members.
c. 8 members.
d. 10 members.

109. If the health impact assessment (HIA) identifies possible adverse health effects resulting from a proposed project, the next action is to:

a. develop recommendations for project changes.
b. discontinue working on the project.
c. conduct a second health impact assessment.
d. develop justification for proceeding as planned.

110. If as part of a cancer prevention program, the health education specialist surveys a group of patients with ovarian cancer to determine what lifestyle choices may have led to development of this form of cancer, this type of study is categorized as:

a. longitudinal.
b. prospective.
c. retrospective.
d. cross-sectional.

111. When providing health education to Native Americans to encourage more use of Western medicine for chronic health problems such as heart disease and diabetes, the best title for the class is probably:

a. Advantage of Western Medicine Over Traditional Native American Healers.
b. Reasons to Avoid Native American Medicine Men/Women.
c. Why Western Medicine Is Safer Than Native American Healing.
d. Combining Western Medicine and Native American Healing.

112. If as part of a needs assessment, the health education specialist is considering the use of an internet survey in order to reduce costs, the health education specialist should first consider:

a. time needed.
b. ease of use.
c. Internet access.
d. secondary costs.

113. The three most important components of the teaching plan are the:

a. purpose, goals, and objectives.
b. purpose, methods, and evaluation.
c. goals, methods, and times.
d. purpose, resources, and methods.

114. When developing a health education program for a large priority population, in order to ensure that community feedback is included, the most effective solution for the health education specialist is:

a. community posters.
b. community advisory board.
c. newspaper requests for input.
d. focus groups.

115. The Plain Writing Act of 2010, which applies to federal agencies, requires that:

a. written communications, such as reports, be in English.
b. reports be written at the fifth grade level.
c. websites be accessible to the disabled.
d. communications be understandable to the average person.

116. If the health education specialist is unsure about the legal standards that may apply to a project, the best solution for the health education specialist is to:

a. consult legal counsel.
b. do further research.
c. ask those with more experience.
d. follow standard procedures.

117. During which stage of change should the health education specialist support the learner's decision making for change by focusing on benefits of change and methods of dealing with obstacles?

a. precontemplation
b. contemplation
c. preparation
d. action

118. In a project that spans a multi-county area with large distances between project members, the best method to use to discuss problems and findings on a weekly basis is probably:

a. meeting in a central location.
b. telephone contact.
c. Dropbox.
d. videoconferencing.

119. If the health education specialist convinces a person to participate in a program that will benefit the person but fails to tell the person everything involved in participation because of the fear the person will not agree, the ethical principle that has been breached is:

a. beneficence.
b. autonomy.
c. equity.
d. justice.

120. With McKenzie et al's five generic phases of program implementation, once a program has been adopted, the next step is to:

a. identify necessary tasks and prioritize them.
b. establish a system of management.
c. activate plans.
d. plan for sustainability.

121. The best way to assess technology needs for a large-scale multi-level program is to:

a. hire a consultant.
b. ask department heads.
c. conduct a survey.
d. ask other program directors.

122. The health education specialist finds that participants routinely do internet searches about their conditions and question every aspect of a risk-reduction program, wanting to assert some control over their choices. This is an example of:

a. consumer advocacy.
b. consumer interference.
c. consumer empowerment.
d. consumer avoidance.

123. If a program is utilizing store-and-forward telehealth technology to monitor clinical data (BP, pulse, ECG), the health education specialist expects:

a. clinical data to be stored on the device and then transmitted at specified times.
b. clinical data to be stored on a memory chip until the device is no longer in use.
c. real-time access to clinical data, which is immediately transmitted.
d. clinical data to be stored on the device permanently.

124. When evaluating a partnership, the health education specialist finds that one partner to the agreement had failed to meet its financial obligations because of unexpected loss of a large grant, forcing the other partner to contribute additional funds to carry out the joint program. The best solution at this point is probably to:

a. disband the partnership.
b. renegotiate the partnership.
c. replace one member of the partnership.
d. form a coalition of other agencies.

125. When developing a logic model to serve as a guide for program development, which of the following should the health education specialist describe first?

a. resources
b. activities
c. expected outcomes
d. impact

126. When identifying evidence to justify a public health program, the best database in which to look for public health data is:

a. The National Library of Medicine.
b. AHRQ.
c. Cochrane Library.
d. CDC Wonder.

127. When designing a communication strategy, the health education specialist carries out a PEST analysis, which looks at the following factors: (P) political, (E) economic, (S) social, and (T):

a. task-oriented.
b. technological
c. testimonial.
d. time-oriented.

128. The health education specialist is working with a priority population of Native Americans to reduce the rates of diabetes and heart disease, but the population tends to eat many foods high in fat, such as fried foods. Because of this, the health education specialist has arranged for a nutritionist to give a series of cooking classes throughout the community to teach people how to lower the fat content of their familiar foods or to use healthier fats. This is an example of:

a. cultural care accommodation.
b. cultural care preservation.
c. cultural care restructuring.
d. cultural care revolution.

129. The health education specialist attends a community meeting and asks a number of the key figures as well as members of the general public unstructured questions about community needs and problems. This type of assessment is referred to as:

a. windshield survey.
b. participant observation.
c. informant interview.
d. random survey.

130. If the people in a Caribbean community tend to believe that illness is caused by supernatural influence, such as evil spirits, this health belief system is referred to as:

a. superstitious.
b. biomedical.
c. humoral.
d. magico-religious.

131. Which of the following is an example of a tertiary intervention at the community level of public health practice?

a. lead screening programs at schools and well-baby clinics
b. environmental cleanup program
c. education about lead poisoning presented at a health fair
d. program to help children with lead exposure–related developmental delay

132. Considering the 4 Ps of social marketing, which is the focus when the health education specialist is considering how information will reach the priority population?

a. product
b. price
c. place
d. promotion

133. The process that commits two or more persons or organizations to reach a common goal by enhancing the capacity of all or one is:

a. collaboration.
b. coalition building.
c. consultation
d. advocacy.

134. Which of the following would be classified as ratio data?

a. type of intervention
b. temperature (Fahrenheit)
c. order of participants finishing a program
d. weight

135. If the health education specialist helps family members to understand their feelings about one family member's schizophrenia, this type of intervention is:

a. cognitive.
b. affective.
c. behavioral.
d. objective.

136. When using the AIDES method in order to improve medication and treatment adherence in a program to enhance the quality of life for older adults with COPD, the steps include:

a. assess, individualize, document, educate, and supervise.
b. advise, illustrate, delegate, employ, and safeguard.
c. accept, identify, demonstrate, enable, and survey.
d. accommodate, institute, diagnose, examine, and strengthen.

137. The health education specialist has implemented a program for post-stroke individuals with aphasia. All of the following are appropriate interventions to aid communication except:

a. provide aids, such as letter boards.
b. be patient.
c. speak slowly and deliberately.
d. praise efforts.

138. Which of the following may be the most effective to aid in research regarding the health effects of air pollution on a priority population in a widespread area?

a. Smart phones
b. GIS technology
c. database program
d. assistive technology

139. The purpose of a culture audit at an organization is to assess the:

a. degree of cultural awareness within an organization.
b. ethnic makeup of the members of an organization.
c. participation of the different members of an organization.
d. overall perceptions and values of an organization.

140. According to Healthy People 2030, *w*hich of the following is a physical determinant of health?

a. access to health services.
b. safe housing.
c. green space.
d. exposure to crime.

141. A community health organization replaces the director and program managers because of a desire to move in a different direction. This approach to change is:

a. revolutionary.
b. evolutionary.
c. punitive.
d. incremental.

142. Which of the following is a concern when considering the need to recruit individuals to fill positions for a program that is in the planning stage?

a. the place that recruitment will occur
b. the type of individual that is appropriate
c. the person(s) who will carry out the recruitment
d. the reason the position is required

Questions 143 and 144 refer to the following information:

Graph 4

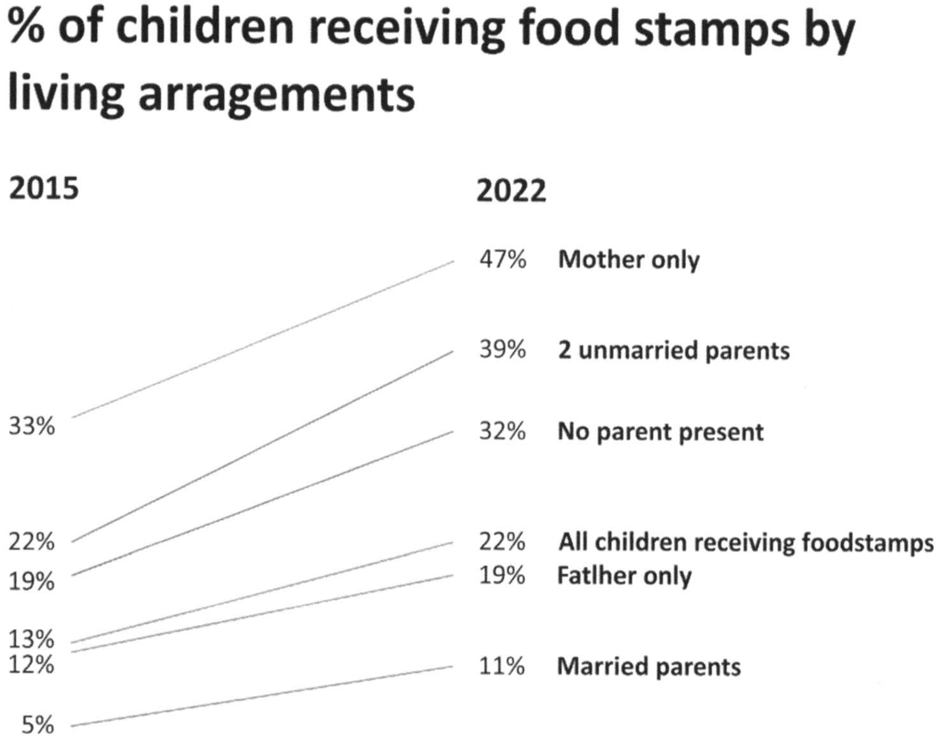

143. When planning an educational program about nutrition for families with limited income, according to the Census Bureau chart for children receiving food stamps (Graph 4), which living situation has resulted in the greatest increase in the percentage of children in need of nutritional assistance?

a. father only
b. two unmarried parents
c. mother only
d. no parent present

144. According to Graph 4, married parents show the least increase in the number of children needing food stamps. This probably reflects the fact that:

a. married parents are actually unmarried but lying.
b. married parents often have higher socioeconomic status.
c. married parents are claiming to be unmarried.
d. data collection was skewed in favor of unmarried individuals.

145. Which of the following would provide the best resource for a health education specialist who is researching measurement tools and instruments?

a. SAMSHA
b. Medline
c. HaPI
d. APA PsychInfo

146. When trying to replicate an evidence-based program for reduction of teen pregnancy, the health education specialist needed to extensively modify some parts of the program in order to meet local policy guidelines and community suitability. Because of this, the health education specialist must also likely modify the:

a. reporting procedures.
b. outcomes evaluation.
c. supervisory functions.
d. time frame for implementation.

147. An individual tells the health education specialist that he is considering controlling his diabetes with a high-protein diet based on information he found in a blog post on the internet. The health education specialist should advise the individual to:

a. follow the blog guidelines.
b. seek information from valid sources.
c. ignore everything he reads online.
d. check the writer's credentials.

148. If the members of a nonprofit agency that conducts a free health clinic want to access information about recommended immunizations for children and adults, the health education specialist should refer them to:

a. CMS.
b. FDA.
c. OSHA.
d. CDC.

149. If the health education specialist is doing research to locate charitable organizations that might donate funds for a suicide prevention program that the health education specialist wants to implement, the best online resource is:

a. Candid.
b. Partnership for Prevention.
c. National Institute of Mental Health (NIMH).
d. Prevention Research Centers.

150. Which of the following is the best choice of a "safe" change to make when preparing evidence-based guidelines for a priority population?

a. Modifying language to reduce medical and technical jargon.
b. Removing statistics and graphs to decrease the amount of material.
c. Condensing the entire guideline from four pages to one.
d. Adding a number of sections based on personal research.

151. When determining what method of presentation to use when sharing information about a program, the first consideration is the:

a. content.
b. audience.
c. time frame.
d. place.

152. A health education specialist who works with four high schools in the county needs to determine what health-related information is most needed by the students. The most efficient method to gain information is:

a. focus groups.
b. interviews with instructors.
c. interviews with students.
d. surveys.

153. The health education specialist must give a presentation to the board of directors of a sponsoring organization. What type of presentation should the health education specialist plan?

a. casual
b. informal
c. formal
d. semiformal

154. A client has been advised to join an exercise program to increase strengthening exercises. According to the Elaboration Likelihood Model of communication, which of the following is an example of the process of persuasion by the central route?

a. The client is confused about the fitness regimen recommended and decides not to bother.
b. The client considers different exercise programs and chooses the one that provides the most benefit.
c. The client joins the most expensive exercise program, assuming it is the best.
d. The client joins an exercise program that has the fanciest equipment and newest facility.

155. The health education specialist is involved in advocacy when the health education specialist:

a. participates in the cleanup of a park along with other community members.
b. believes that it is necessary to clean up the park to encourage children to exercise.
c. votes against politicians who have refused to provide funds to clean up the park.
d. addresses the county board of supervisors about the importance of cleaning up a park.

156. Which of the following is an independent accreditation agency for public health services?

a. WASC
b. PHAB
c. SACS
d. CAEP

157. Resource materials obtained from an online site should be evaluated for (1) accuracy, (2) relevance, and (3):

a. replication.
b. clarity.
c. authority.
d. timeliness.

158. When assessing literacy, if a client is able to read and understand a consent form, according to the National Adult Literacy Survey categorizations, the person is said to have literacy related to:

a. document tasks.
b. prose tasks.
c. quantitative tasks.
d. qualitative tasks.

159. If, as part of an educational program, the health education specialist is designing a website that includes a message board where clients can discuss their progress, the primary concern is:

a. the cost of maintaining the message board.
b. the need to monitor the message board.
c. the need to instruct clients in use of the message board.
d. the need to develop rules of use for the message board.

160. When planning a media campaign to promote a program, which of the following is likely to have the largest audience reach?

a. Radio
b. Internet
c. Television
d. Newspaper

161. When conducting community-based teaching with older learners, it is best to limit sessions to:

a. 10-15 minutes.
b. 20-30 minutes.
c. 30-45 minutes.
d. 45-60 minutes.

162. The five elements of an advocacy plan are (1) goals, (2) organizational considerations, (3) constituents, allies, and opponents, (4) targets, and (5):

a. tactics.
b. finances.
c. timeliness.
d. communication.

163. When selecting an instrument for data collection, the first questions to ask is:

a. "Is the instrument at the appropriate readability level?"
b. "How difficult is it to administer the instrument?"
c. "Is the instrument well written and constructed?"
d. "Does the instrument measure the correct data?"

164. If the object of data collection is to assess patterns of discharge from a healthcare facility, the best initial method is probably:

a. surveys.
b. record review.
c. interviews.
d. focus group.

165. Facebook, LinkedIn, Twitter, and SnapChat are used to market an educational program. These are examples of:

a. broadcast media.
b. social media.
c. print media.
d. modern media.

Answer Key and Explanations for Test #1

1. C: If advising members of the general public about the most valid online source for health information, the health education specialist should advise them to look for URLs that end with .gov. Many organizations (.org) are valid sources, such as the American Heart Association (heart.org), but there are millions of organizations and not all provide valid information. While educational URLs (.edu) may contain valid information, some institutions provide the URL to all students, so the author's credentials must be checked.

2. A: If a client has enrolled in a program to reduce obesity but not lost weight because he or she did not stay on the diet or exercise program, and then concludes the program is not effective because of the failure to lose weight, this exemplifies the cognitive dissonance theory of communication. Cognitive dissonance refers to the tension that develops when a person must make a choice. The mind attempts to attain harmony and reduce tension by changing attitudes or behavior or rationalizing behavior in order to justify choices.

3. C: If a health education specialist working in the public health field wants to become active in a professional organization, the Society for Public Health Education (SOPHE) may best serve the health education specialist's needs. SOPHE establishes yearly health priorities for advocacy and publishes numerous books and three peer-reviewed journals about public health issues. SOPHE also provides continuing education courses as well as a number of programs and initiatives. Members can access 13 different online communities.

4. D: If the health education specialist is interested in using an asset-based community development strategy to implement a program, the first step is to map capacities and assets of all elements of the priority population, including individuals, organizations, and institutions. Asset-based community development looks to the strengths of a community and tries to identify and use those strengths for program development, building partnerships and coalitions, and developing a consensus about vision, mission, and objectives.

5. B: In order to be effective, implementation of a program of blood pressure screening and treatment should include lifestyle counseling, usually presented as one-on-one education so that the individual with elevated blood pressure can develop a plan to reduce risk factors, such as smoking and obesity. The lifestyle counseling may be provided by members of the program or may be a benefit included in the individual's insurance coverage, although many will not take advantage of this benefit without encouragement.

6. C: While all of these are important, the best preparation for total implementation of a program is usually pilot testing, a small-scale preliminary testing, because it is often easier to identify problems that may arise on a small scale and to fix those problems than to try to deal with them on a larger scale. Pilot testing should be carried out in a self-contained area if possible so that the testing does not impact others.

7. A: The Boolean operator *OR* is used to locate synonymous terms or concepts, such as "stroke" or "CVA." There are only three Boolean operators: AND, OR, and NOT. These operators are almost always capitalized. When AND, which is restrictive, is used between terms, then any document retrieved must contain both terms. The Boolean term NOT is also restrictive and is used to eliminate concepts so that a document retrieved contains one term but not another.

8. D: Hotline counseling is an example of an interpersonal channel of communication. Other interpersonal activities include counseling patients, individual instruction, informal discussion, fact sheets with questions to ask healthcare providers, guidebooks, and videos to promote discussion. The interpersonal channel allows two-way discussion and may be effective in teaching. The interpersonal channel also allows the message to be geared to the culture of the participant. However, the use of the interpersonal channel can be costly and time intensive and has limited audience reach.

9. C: If utilizing the Critical Path Method work plan, the step that must be completed first is to identify activities that will be required. The next step is to organize these in chronological order (identifying predecessors—activities that should be completed before another activity can begin) and to estimate time for each activity. Some activities may be carried out concurrently. An activity-on-arc (ARC) diagram is used with the nodes (activities) numbered and arrows connecting them. The diagram should clearly show predecessors.

10. A: NIDDK (National Institute of Diabetes and Digestive and Kidney Diseases), which is part of the National Institutes of Health, can provide the most extensive information about diabetes mellitus. NIDDK includes research and funding in the form of grants as well as health information regarding health topics, clinical trials, health statistics, and clinical outreach. NIDDK provides links to news releases and a multimedia gallery. NIDDK provides information both for healthcare providers and consumers.

11. B: Based on Graph 1, since 2005 the birthrate among unmarried women ages 18-44 in the United States has decreased. A line graph with multiple lines is an excellent way to demonstrate comparative ordinal data and trends. Line graphs have an *X* axis and a *Y* axis and can have a secondary *X* and/or *Y* axis as well, as in this case with two X axes, one indicating percentages of births per 1000 unmarried women and the other indicating births in thousands. Lines should be in different shades or colors to help to differentiate them, especially if the lines run close together or cross.

12. D: According to Graph 1, the decade in which the number of births to unmarried women increased the most was 1980-1990, increasing from approximately 750-1250 births. The increase in births was steady but slow from about 1950-1975, and then the number of births began to increase markedly as the stigma associated with having children out of wedlock eased. The highest rates were at about 2005, but the rates have shown a decrease since then, possibly reflecting decreasing rates of teenage pregnancy.

13. A: Under the HIPAA privacy rule, health information may be used for research purposes without patient authorization if it is de-identified; that is, information that could be used to identify the person has been removed, such as name, birthdate, or ID number. The privacy rule allows researchers to use individually identifiable information with individual authorization or when the IRB or privacy board has approved a waiver of authorization. The privacy rule also states requirements for the individual to be informed about use and disclosure of medical information.

14. B: While severe anxiety often clearly hinders the acquisition of skills, moderate anxiety actually has a positive effect because it causes the person to take action and to concentrate. If a person is only mildly anxious, this can lead to apathy and inaction. Factors that can hinder the acquisition of skills include lack of motivation; complexity of the skills involved in the task; and environmental effects, such as noise, interruptions, or inadequate lighting.

15. B: The most effective method of teaching participants in a program the technical skills needed to utilize electronic equipment is hands-on practice, often presented as just-in-time instruction so that the participants have practice at the time that they need to master a particular skill. Trial and error is usually the least effective method of learning skills and can result in wasted time and mistakes. Video guides may be useful as preparation or as review, and written manuals should be available as a reference.

16. C: When completing a review of literature as part of quantitative research, the review of literature should be carried out at the beginning of the research process. The review is a critical element in developing and implementing a study. Further review may also be conducted at a later point in the research, depending on the results of the study. In quantitative research, sources that result from the literature review are usually cited in multiple sections of the research document: the introduction, the methods, the results, and the discussion.

17. D: When carrying out a critical appraisal of a quantitative study, the first step in determining the validity of a quantitative study is comprehension. The health education specialist must have an understanding of the terms and concepts utilized in the study in order to accurately assess validity. The health education specialist should begin by reading the abstract and researching any unfamiliar terms. After reading the study, the health education specialist should be able to outline the steps to the research process and to summarize the results of the study.

18. A: While all of these factors—consistency, time frame, costs, and attitude—are important when training personnel to assist with data collection, consistency is the most critical. Data that are collected in a different manner may skew the findings, may be difficult to evaluate, or may be unusable. The personnel should be provided data collection forms and receive training in exactly how to obtain and record the data. The personnel should have practice time, and collected data should be periodically assessed for consistency.

19. B: The four primary tasks in data collection are:

1. Selecting subjects: This is the first task. Subjects may be selected randomly from a population or may include a specific group or population according to preselected criteria.
2. Collecting data systematically: A procedure should be outlined and data collection forms created.
3. Maintaining research controls: Data collection should be evaluated for consistency and accuracy.
4. Solving problems: Problems that arise should be dealt with as quickly and efficiently as possible.

20. C: Advocacy evaluation should be considered during the planning stages of an advocacy program. As the goals of the advocacy program are outlined, the methods of assessing outcomes should be built into the plan as well as the time frame for evaluation and the method of disseminating the results of the evaluation. The Innovation Network (Innonet.org) is a free clearinghouse that provides advocacy evaluation resources and can provide valuable information regarding evaluation.

21. C: While there is value in reading about the target population, applying general educational principles, and asking other health education specialists for advice, if the health education specialist must create an educational program for an immigrant group with whom the health education specialist is not familiar, the best approach is to interview some members of that community. This is a good way to begin to establish a relationship with the immigrant group and to find out more about the people's culture and their specific needs.

22. B: Because Mexican culture is male dominated, the father in a family of immigrants is usually the ultimate authority and likely to be the one to make a decision about participating in interviews or other activities, so it is important to address the father and to show respect for the family's traditions. Mexicans tend to be very family oriented and often live with or near other family members, whom they may consult. Catholicism is the primary religion of Mexican immigrants, and some people may consult a priest about decisions.

23. B: The strategy that is used when replacing sugar-laden drinks in vending machines with juice or sugar-free drinks is health engineering in which changes are made to effect improvement in health. Health engineering involves making changes that may affect large populations. The changes may be in the social and/or physical environment. The focus may be on safety issues, such as consumer product safety, or social issues, such as improving access to public transportation.

24. C: If a potential research subject is led to believe that the individual's medical care will be adversely affected if the individual does not participate in a research project, this is an example of *coercion*. Essentially, the person is forced to participate because of fear. Coercion may also involve a direct threat or a promise of some type of reward in exchange for participation. However, small amounts of money offered to pay expenses, such as transportation costs, are not considered coercive.

25. A: When collecting data in the community about substance abuse and comparing it with national data, a good secondary source of data is the Substance Abuse and Mental Health Services Administration (SAMHSA). Primary data are those that the researcher collects, such as through surveys and interviews, while secondary data are those that are collected by others, such as government agencies. Secondary data are usually available free of cost or for minimal cost. Secondary data are especially valuable for comparative data.

26. C: If a needs assessment includes the observation that local health clinics are serving large numbers of pregnant adolescents, the type of need this represents is expressed. Expressed needs are those that can be inferred through observation of trends within a community. Expressed needs must be carefully assessed, as it is easy to misinterpret observations. For example, an increased demand for service at one health clinic may actually represent increased need or it may represent lack of alternative resources.

27. D: Increased exposure to mass media is a social determinant that can impact health, both negatively (such as the anti-immunization campaign) and positively. Other social determinants include educational opportunities, employment opportunities, and discrimination. Socioeconomic factors also impact health, including not only income but also transportation options, and levels of crime within a neighborhood or community. Physical determinants, such as the environment, type of housing, exposure to toxins, and lighting, also affect health.

28. B: The place of residence is likely to have the least influence on health behaviors. While this may seem counterintuitive, especially considering people who are homeless or live in substandard housing, the bigger issue that affects health behavior is socioeconomic status (which may be reflected in the place of residence). Race also has less influence on health behavior than other factors, such as age (both young and advanced), gender, and social support network.

29. A: The legalization of marijuana may have the most influence on health not only for adverse effects associated with recreational use but also for positive effects associated with medical uses.

Medical marijuana is used to treat a wide variety of ailments, including pain, nausea (especially associated with chemotherapy), muscle spasms (associated with multiple sclerosis), Crohn disease, and seizure disorders. In some cases, an active ingredient in marijuana (THC), which is FDA approved, may be prescribed for nausea and to improve appetite.

30. D: There are usually no financial and only limited time costs associated with the use of secondary data, as much of the data are easily available online. However, secondary data may, in some cases, be too broad, but the data are of value for demographic and comparison purposes. Surveys, whether online or on paper, are relatively inexpensive for small groups. If large populations are to be surveyed and paper surveys must be mailed, then postage costs can be quite high. Interviews require considerable time and sometimes expense.

31. C: When developing a vision statement, the vision should focus on future goals—where the organization wants to be at a future time rather than the current status. Vision statements usually comprise one sentence or a short paragraph but may be followed by explanation of terms to help clarify the goals of the vision statement. The vision statement should be based on assessment and should be stated clearly so that people can develop strategies in support of the vision.

32. A: Histograms are most often used to display continuous data. A histogram is similar to a bar chart but there is no space between the bars. The histogram has both an *X* and *Y* axis, which should be labeled, with the *X* axis on the horizontal scale and the *Y* on the vertical. Categorical data, which are distinct groups without overlap, may be displayed in a number of different ways, such as with a pie chart, line graph, or bar graph.

33. D: Emotional readiness to learn is most affected by motivation. People who want to learn or see the benefit in learning are more likely to be invested in the learning process. Other factors that affect emotional readiness include the person's level of anxiety, the support system available to the person, risk-taking behavior, and the person's frame of mind and developmental stage. Other types of readiness to learn include physical readiness, experiential readiness, and knowledge readiness.

34. C: If the health education specialist regularly communicates directions and status updates to staff members regarding a program being implemented in the form of read-only e-mails, the primary problem with this form of communication is that it is one-way. It is important to avoid one-way vertical or horizontal communication as this type of communication suggests the message sender is not interested in the ideas of others, and this can prevent people from making valuable contributions.

35. B: If the health education specialist wants to begin an advocacy campaign to increase the number of shelters for the homeless in order to reduce illness and injury among the homeless population, the first step is to gather allies and supporters. While one person can advocate, there is strength in numbers, and large numbers of people are more likely to get results. The health education specialist may develop a power grid that shows the agencies or organizations with sufficient power to help the cause.

36. D: In the objective, "Following a class on HIV prevention, the participants will be able to describe transmission," the criterion for mastery is inadequate because it is vague and not measurable. The condition/testing situation (following a class on HIV prevention) is followed by a description of the learners (the participants) and the performance (will be able to). The criterion for mastery must be more specific (describe at least 5 methods of transmission).

37. C: If a needs assessment indicates a need for a program within the community to combat childhood obesity, the resource that is probably most critical is financial. While environmental support is probably not essential, and social support may be garnered through educational efforts and marketing, developing a program almost always entails additional costs. In some cases, political support may be necessary to gain necessary funds, but often funds must be taken from an existing budget or received from a grant following an application process.

38. A: When prioritizing needs for health education, the first step is to identify criteria, usually at least two, such as cost and impact or importance and feasibility. Then, the proposals are evaluated based on the pre-established criteria. If, for example, financial resources are limited, then cost may be the primary criterion, so any proposals that require additional funds could be eliminated unless alternate sources of funding can be identified. Strategy grids may be utilized to help determine the proposal with the highest priority.

39. C: A goal statement should state the desired end result rather than the process, so an appropriate goal statement is: "Lower the cost of health care through prevention strategies." The goal represents the ideal that may be reached in the future. The objectives, then, would be the steps taken to reach this goal, such as providing classes in smoking cessation, providing emergency shelter for the homeless, and teaching parents strategies to prevent childhood obesity.

40. A: Based on the Graph 2 showing contraceptive use among sexually active females at a university, approximately 15% of females use both a condom and another form of birth control. Since 50% of the females use condoms and 40% use other forms of birth control (diaphragms, pills, injectables, and IUD/implants), this equals 90% of the students. Since 25% use no birth control at all, that leaves only 75% using birth control. The difference between 90% and 75% is 15%, which is the percentage of the females who appear to be using two forms of birth control.

41. A: When developing an education plan for university students about safe sex, the health education specialist should consider all students to be the priority population. Although Graph 2 depicts contraceptive use among sexually active females, males are equally at risk with unsafe sex practices, and only 50% of sexually active females use a condom for contraception or protection, and other forms of contraception provide no protection against sexually transmitted diseases. Additionally, females often expect males to provide condoms and do not do so themselves.

42. D: The level of education is a demographic factor that may be considered when identifying a priority population. Other demographic factors include age, gender, race/ethnicity, level of income, marital status, and health status. Geographic factors, such as the community or state of residence, may also be used to identify a population. In some cases, a priority population may be identified by location, such as attendance at a particular school, church, or organization.

43. C: If the health education specialist is a member of an advocacy group trying to develop a halfway house for substance abusers in a neighborhood and is confronted by people who are adamantly opposed to the project, the best initial response is to determine the reason for the opposition through both dialog and investigation. People may have valid concerns that need to be voiced, and those in opposition are more likely to alter their stance if their opinions are respected.

44. B: When eliciting input about a health education plan for a priority population, input that is most critical usually comes from the priority population itself. The success of an education plan often depends on the commitment of the population to participate, and engaging this population in the formation of the project and allowing the people to express their needs and concerns can motivate participation. It is important that education programs not appear to be imposed on a population.

45. A: When a number of different advocacy groups are all focused on one goal or issue, such as improving women's health, this is an example of a community of ideas. If advocacy groups respond to a crisis, such as a marked increase in heroin addiction and overdose, these groups form a community of crisis. If advocacy groups work toward legal status for illegal immigrants, they may form a community of memory because of shared experiences over a period of time.

46. C: When designing interventions to reduce risk-taking behavior in a population, the ethical principle that is applied when participants are assured that use of illicit drugs will not be reported to the police is *confidentiality*. Confidentiality is especially important when dealing with risk-taking behaviors, which are often viewed negatively by others, because participants are not likely to cooperate if they fear punishment. Terms of confidentiality should be clearly spelled out so that participants understand the circumstances in which confidentiality may be breached.

47. A: When planning an outreach program for the homeless community, the best place to provide information about the program to people who are homeless and may benefit is likely shelters and soup kitchens. Contacting people on the street may be difficult because they are often scattered throughout a community. The homeless may avoid churches and community centers unless they have programs specifically for the homeless because of fear that they are not wanted or welcome, or because of shame.

48. B: The best way to ensure a commitment to participate in an educational program is to assist people to pre-register. People are more likely to participate if they have taken an official step, such as signing up or pre-registering. While charging a fee may ensure commitment, it may also have the opposite effect of deterring people from committing to the program, especially low-income populations. Asking people to commit or sending out literature asking for phone registration has lower results than one-on-one interaction.

49. D: When searching for a facility in which to hold classes for a priority population, the first consideration should be ADA compliance. The room should be wheelchair accessible, which means ramps and/or elevators should be available. According to ADA regulations, the first priority is accessibility of the approach and entrance of the building. The second priority is access to goods and services. The third is access to restrooms, and the fourth is other necessary measures.

50. C: If the goal is to encourage active participation among all class members, the best seating arrangement for a group of 10 participants is in a circle. This configuration allows all members of the group see each other during discussions and makes the leader appear more as part of the group rather than the authoritarian. Additionally, if participants are sitting in a circle, it is easier to draw out participants who usually sit at the back of the room or avoid participation.

51. B: Media advocacy involves a number of different activities, including writing op-ed articles for local newspapers or letters to the editor at various media outlets, including those that target specific ethnic groups. Video productions using Flash or animation software can be posted on internet sites, such as an organization's website or on YouTube. Media advocacy can include calling in to radio to discuss a topic as well as recording interviews. The health education specialist should frame narratives in such a way as to garner interest, such as pointing out controversy or areas of specific concern.

52. A: For a slide presentation (such as with PowerPoint) that is to accompany a lecture, a well-designed presentation should not contain the complete lecture text but only highlights, preferably with one or two points per slide. Learners tend to read the text on the slides and ignore the presenter, so the text should remain limited with san serif font used for text because it is easier to read. Showing illustrations and diagrams is a good use of slides and can save narrative time.

53. D: If the health education specialist has conducted a media campaign to increase HPV vaccinations of both boys and girls at two local clinics, the best method to evaluate the impact is to monitor the number of vaccinations provided. The health education specialist may choose a time period of 1-2 months or longer and can compare the number of HPV vaccinations during this time period with the same time period in the previous year or years.

54. D: Determining whether an education program was worth the investment and should be continued is part of impact evaluation. Impact is usually done at a later time than summative evaluation, which assesses the effect teaching has had on outcomes. Impact evaluation tries to determine the overall effect or impact the program has had, so the scope of the evaluation is usually broader and more comprehensive than other forms of evaluation.

55. C: PRECEDE, which has 3 phases (1-3), is an acronym for Predisposing, Reinforcing, and Enabling Constructs in Educational/Environmental Diagnosis and Evaluation, and is done as part of the assessment leading up to a project or intervention. In phase 1, social assessment is carried out to define the priority population's quality of life. PROCEED, which has an additional 5 phases (4-8), is an acronym for Policy, Regulatory, and Organizational Constructs in Educational and Environmental Development.

56. A: If the health education specialist is involved in an advocacy group with a national focus, the best way to gain local supporters is to focus on local issues that are related to the national issue. For example, if the national issue is to have stricter punishment for drunk driving in order to reduce injuries and fatalities, the health education specialist should address statistics regarding drunk driving in the community and injuries or fatalities that have resulted.

57. D: If the leaders from two partnered agencies meet and attempt together to determine how to divide up grant money to best meet the financial needs of both agencies, the negotiation style is collaborative because the aim is to satisfy both needs. The competitive style usually involves a winning side and a losing side. The accommodative style of negotiation involves one side making concessions, while the compromising style usually involves concessions on both sides.

58. A: When two agencies form a partnership, the type of resource that the partnership itself represents is intellectual because the partnership is intangible. Intellectual resources may also include knowledge, skills, and agreements. Intellectual resources may lead to other types of resources, such as financial or physical, if utilized properly. Intellectual resources are often the most critical elements in a program development and are directly related to human resources, making the appropriate selection of key participants crucial to success.

59. C: If the health education specialist is assessing the types of problems that developed in the implementation of a program and whether the resources and training were adequate to achieve the desired results, this is an example of process evaluation. Process evaluations assess the interventions, including how they are carried out and how successful they are as well as the types of problems that arise and the steps carried out to manage the problems.

60. B: When planning learning assignments, the health education specialist should realize that the least retention is likely to occur with reading because people usually retain only about 10%. Listening to information results in 20% retention, while seeing, such as from watching a demonstration, 30%. When seeing and listening are combined, the sum is greater than the parts with 50% retention, but people retain 70% of that which they say, and 90% of that which they do (such as through practice) and say (such as by restating or teaching others).

61. A: If giving a presentation to a community group about the results of a health prevention strategy, the best method to convey the statistical changes is likely a line chart. The line chart shows changes visually in an easy to understand format. While a table may hold the same information, it does not allow people to visualize the changes and is more difficult to interpret. Narratives may be confusing or misunderstood. Raw data requires interpretation that may be difficult for some participants.

62. D: While addressing different learning styles, presenting information that is easily accessible by the learners and assessing costs are important when evaluating instructional methods, the most important issue is whether the method helps learners achieve goals and objectives. Even though satisfaction with the instruction may be high, the instruction is ineffective if the learners do not learn what was intended. If this occurs, then the health education specialist must consider that the methods of instruction and the lesson plans may require modification to better support the goals and objectives.

63. B: Immigrant populations are often wary of officials and reluctant to allow strangers into their homes, and may be distrustful about the offer of free smoke and carbon monoxide alarms. The best solution is to offer free alarms and instructions at community gathering places, such as churches and social clubs. Information and instructions should be in both English and the immigrant's first language. Video presentations that show placement of the alarms are especially valuable.

64. A: A typical logic model contains:

1. Inputs: various types of resources (human, financial, physical) required to develop goals and objectives
2. Activities: activities planned with available resources resulting in measurable objectives
3. Outputs: products, services, and activities that are produced and can influence short-term outcomes
4. Outcomes/Impacts: changes in behavior, knowledge, skills, morbidity, and mortality that result from interventions; may be short-term, intermediate, or long-term

65. C: Pilot studies are used for a number of reasons, but a pilot study is unlikely to assess for long-term outcomes. Some of the primary purposes of a pilot study are to determine feasibility, to guide modifications, and to examine reliability, validity, and usability. The pilot study allows testing of instruments, training, education, or other interventions, and can help to determine if explanations are sufficient. The pilot study may also result in unanticipated results or findings, and this information may be critical to success or failure.

66. B: The factor that is most likely to foster implementation of an educational program is community support. Regardless of the marketing plan, legislative guidelines, and media support (which are also important), the program is unlikely to succeed if the community members that are targeted by the program are not supportive. For this reason, it is important to include community members in the planning phases so that they do not feel that the program is imposed upon them.

67. A: While all who observe a staff member being physically abusive to an adolescent in a program have a moral obligation to report physical abuse to the authorities, the social worker is a mandated reporter and is required by law to do so. While state laws vary somewhat as to who is a mandated reporter and to whom the person should report, in most cases abuse is reported to child protective services or adult protective services, depending on the age of the victim.

68. C: *Skill inoculation* refers to repeated practice of tasks, but this practice does not always have to be hands-on practice, although this is preferable. Skill inoculation can also include providing reminders about the task, reviewing previously studies or learned material, and return demonstration. The health education specialist should provide as many opportunities for skill inoculation as possible when planning lessons because repetition reinforces learning and moves information from short-term memory to long-term memory.

69. D: If developing a substance abuse program for homeless veterans in a residential community where residents have resisted such programs in the past, the health education specialist should notify the residents in advance. To fail to do so would be unethical, even though the residents may take legal actions to try to halt the program, such as by filing a civil suit. The notification should provide not only information about the program but also the rationale for locating it within the community and the benefits that the community may derive from the program.

70. C: Prior to beginning the first phase of implementation of a new program, the health education specialist should review the program budget. While some of the budget may have been utilized during the planning phase and the budget for implementation developed in advance, changes may have occurred that will affect costs. If funds are not adequate for complete implementation, then alternate sources of funds must be found or the program must be scaled back or phased in.

71. B: When recruiting individuals needed for implementation of an education plan, the health education specialist should first develop a job description. The description should be detailed and include all duties. The interview questions should be developed after the job description so that questions can be directed toward the skills needed. The salary may be predetermined but should be reviewed in relation to the job description and the responsibilities of the position. While personal characteristics may be important, focusing on these when recruiting individuals may lead to bias.

72. C: When collecting baseline data prior to implementation of a program, the first place to begin is usually secondary data collection. The demographic information that is often available may provide a benchmark against which primary data can be evaluated. In some cases, other agencies or organizations may have already obtained the necessary data, precluding the need for primary data collection by the health education specialist. Baseline information is critical for eventual evaluation of outcomes.

73. A: The first step in securing resources to implement a plan is to identify the resources needed. This list should then be reviewed in relation to the budgetary allowances for resources to determine if funds are adequate. If not, alternate sources of funds must be identified or the list modified. Then, any existing resources, such as personnel and equipment, should be accounted for, and potential sources of resources should be identified.

74. D: If searching a database for lists of journal articles in the field of biomedics, the best resource is MEDLINE, which is a bibliographic database provided by the US National Library of Medicine (NLM). MEDLINE is a component of PubMed. MEDLINE provides listings of journals as well as some newspapers and magazines. In some cases, links to full-text articles in PubMed Central are available. If an article is not available online, a link for ordering the article is provided.

75. C: When conducting a survey, the type of questions that are most difficult to quantify are open-ended because every participant in the survey may write a different answer or may use different words to describe essentially the same thing, requiring subjective assessment on the part of the researcher. Open-ended questions may provide qualitative information. Questions in which the responses can be counted, such as true/false, multiple choice, and rating scale, can be easily quantified.

76. B: When using a Program Evaluation and Review Technique (PERT) chart for time management, the three time estimates that should be included for each activity are optimistic (the best-case scenario), likely (most probable), and pessimistic (worst case scenario). Using these time estimates, the expected time can be calculated:

$$(\text{Optimistic} + 4\text{x likely} + \text{pessimistic}) \div 6 = \text{expected time}$$

So, if the optimistic time is 8 weeks, the likely 9, and the pessimistic 12:

$$8 + 36 + 12 = 56 \div 6 = 9.3 \text{ expected weeks}$$

77. D: Organizational readiness for implementation is exemplified by commitment to change, ability to bring about change, and positive attitude toward change. While establishment of a timeline for implementation is an important step, if the organization has not exhibited readiness, the timeline is not likely to change that important factor. The health education specialist must take an active role in contacting key stakeholders and garnering support for implementation in order to facilitate capacity building.

78. A: If a pop-up message promoting a health program appears on an individual's computer screen based on the individual's browsing history of gyms, weight loss programs, and health-related sites, this is an example of a tailored message because it is specifically tailored to the individual's interests. Websites use cookies to track individual's interests and may sell this information to other sites. Tailored messages are often disseminated through newsletters, pamphlets, mail, and social media.

79. C: If a health education program that was presented in group classes is to be updated so the material can be presented on the internet, the most cost-effective approach is generally to assess, modify, and use existing materials. For example, the basic course outline may remain unchanged, and slide show presentations used in class may be used as part of the internet presentation. Scanning and using materials without modification is a poor strategy and may be initially cost-saving but not cost-effective in the long-run if the number of participants is low or dropout is high.

80. D: If utilizing the social-ecological model when developing preventive strategies, the first level focuses on the individual, including factors (personal, biological) that may increase risk to the individual. Preventive efforts focus on education and training to modify behavior. The second level focuses on relationships (peers, family, neighbors), while the third level focuses on the characteristics of settings in the community (schools, churches, job sites) that may influence behavior and contribute to or solve problems. The fourth level focuses on social factors in a broad context, including cultural norms.

81. A: If a recent outbreak of severe nausea and vomiting has been traced to use of a banned pesticide in fruit orchards, and the health education specialist must develop an educational campaign to warn the public, the first step in identifying the priority population is to study the distribution of cases and demographic information. This is used to determine if there are patterns that may emerge, such as environmental clusters or specific age or cultural groups that are most affected.

82. B: If developing an educational program based on evidence-based research and using the RE-AIM method to improve generalizability and sustainability, the first issue to consider is <u>reaching</u> the priority population. The next step is to question the effectiveness of interventions and measures to evaluate outcomes. The following step is to consider support for adoption. This is followed by consideration of implementation and methods of ensuring that the program is implemented properly. The last step to consider is maintenance and issues of sustainability.

83. C: While cost-effectiveness, community support, and ease of use are important, when choosing materials/interventions for an education program, the most important consideration is that the materials/interventions be evidence based. It is almost always easier and less expensive to use materials and processes that have already been validated and proven to be effective through outcomes assessment than to develop new materials or interventions. The processes involved in determining the validity, reliability, usability, and generalizability of materials/interventions can be both costly and lengthy.

84. D: In order to adequately evaluate the outcomes of interventions, it is necessary that there be intervention fidelity. That is, the interventions should be consistently carried out in the same manner. If intervention fidelity is lacking, then an assessment of outcomes lacks not only internal validity and but also external validity by extension. Those utilizing interventions must be adequately trained and should have an implementation manual that clearly outlines procedures in order to avoid variance.

85. B: Based on the information in Graph 3, people in the Northeast are more likely to consult a psychiatrist for mental illness–related physician visits than a primary care physician or other physician. According to the graph, approximately 65% of people seeking help in the Northeast are seen by a psychiatrist while about 25% are seen by a primary care physician and 10% by another type of physician, a 30% difference. In other parts of the country, there is very little difference in the number seeing psychiatrists and the number seeing primary care or other physicians.

86. A: "By 2025, pregnancy rates of adolescents in the Sandcity community will decrease by 50%," is an example of an impact objective because it shows the long-term results of interventions. Process objectives, such as, "By June 2023, the health education specialist will have conducted 6 classes regarding preventing pregnancy for adolescents at the local high schools and community center," involve the actions that will be undertaken to bring about outcome objectives, such as,, "By June 2023, surveys of adolescents in the Sandcity community will indicate a 25% increase in the use of condoms," and, "By June 2023, at least 80% of adolescents who were provided literature are aware of the need to practice birth control."

87. B: The finding that organization members lack understanding of organizational vision represents a need for increased capacity because the organization is deficient in a key factor. A capacity assessment reviews the levels of capacity and may look at the present situation, for example, or at the last year or previous years, and should address different types of capacity, such as resources and leadership qualities. The assessment should begin with a clear definition of capacity and an understanding of the purpose of the assessment and its relationship to organizational goals.

88. C: The most important aspect of a training program is usually the instructor's ability. While the setting, equipment, and time of instruction may have an impact, positive or negative, on training, the ability of the instructor to communicate well and to utilize strategies that engage the participants is a critical factor. The quality of instruction is often more important than the method utilized. The instructor should be knowledgeable and prepared for each session and should find ways to keep participants interested.

89. A: When developing a marketing plan, the first element to consider is the priority population in order to determine the best means of communicating with this group. While a marketing strategy may be inexpensive, if it fails to reach the priority population, then the money spent on the marketing has been wasted. Program development should include surveys, interviews, and/or focus groups in order to assess characteristics of the priority population in order to better deliver a program tailored to their needs and to identify the best marketing plan.

90. D: A printed case study is an example of a low-fidelity simulation used for educational purposes. Low-fidelity simulations are relatively inexpensive and easy to develop. Low-fidelity simulations include verbal presentations, printed materials, or audio descriptions, and are often used to promote or supplement discussions. However, low-fidelity simulations may be inadequate to teach the use of equipment. High-fidelity simulations include materials that are actual (such as AEDs and blood pressure cuffs) or realistic (such as mannequins).

91. B: If developing podcasts for a community education program, the health education specialist should limit the length to about 10 minutes as studies show that people begin to lose interest after about 10-15 minutes. Thus, it is better to divide a topic into two parts if it requires a longer time. The health education specialist should plan the podcasts carefully, writing a script and practicing before the final recording. Podcasts can be accessed on computers and various hand-held devices (tablets, smart phones, iPods) and have the advantage of portability.

92. C: When a health education specialist is making decisions about how to transmit information to individuals in an education program, this is utilizing communicative decision making because the focus is on the mode of communication. Targeted decision making involves a decision identifying the priority population. Informative decision making involves a decision to seek information in order to increase knowledge of a subject. Preventive decision making involves making a decision that will provide a positive outcome rather than a negative one.

93. D: Aggregate data include demographic information, such as age, gender, and ethnicity, and encompasses financial or budgetary information, information about hazards or safety, as well as business reports and business transactions. Aggregate data is combined data, usually from a large number of different sources. Aggregation allows the combined data to be easily summarized so that patterns can be detected. Aggregate data cannot provide information about an individual but only about groups of individuals.

94. A: Placing ads on television about a community program to reduce drinking and driving and to provide free rides to impaired individuals is an example of using paid media. Paid media may also include ads on the radio or in print or digital form. While television stations and other media outlets may run ads as a public service announcement without cost, these free ads often run in the morning or very late at night rather than during primetime when more people are watching television.

95. B: If an educational program at an organization is to be successful, it is most important to have management support. Management usually controls the resources needed for the program, and these may be important for a viable program. More importantly, management sets the tone of an organization. The audience for the program is more likely to be receptive to participation if management has been proactive and positive in promoting the program and describing benefits of participation as this promotes an environment conducive to learning.

96. A: In addition to financial support, space, and curriculum, resources critical to implementation of an education plan include personnel to help implement the program and supplies and equipment needed. Without these 5 resources, implementation of an education plan may be difficult or impossible. The health education specialist must determine how much or how many of each resource is needed, and he or she may need to use creative approaches to obtain the necessary resources.

97. D: If two nonprofit community agencies have agreed to implement a joint project and create a memorandum of understanding (MOU), the first section of the MOU should contain the intent of the project, explaining what the parties will do. The next sections should describe the parties and the types of organizations. The time period should be specified with starting date and ending date (or open date if the program is to be ongoing). The responsibilities for each party should be clearly outlined as well as any disclaimers, financial arrangements, and risk-sharing elements.

98. C: If the work plan and timeline show that implementation is far behind schedule and the health education specialist plans to modify the implementation plan, he or she must assess the effect that modification will have on fidelity. The outcomes should be unaffected by any modification. Modification can bring about unexpected results and may, in fact, alter the program in ways that are unintended. The health education specialist should carefully assess the reasons for the delay in implementation.

99. A: If, as part of a health-related strategy, policies are enacted to discourage alcohol/substance misuse and institute a drug-free workplace, the first step in implementation is publishing the drug-free policy. Worker must have a clear understanding of the policy and what it means if an individual does not conform to the policy. Subsequently, the staff must be educated about alcohol/substance abuse and provided tools for self-assessment. An employee assistance program (EAP) that ensures privacy for those seeking treatment should be available for referral.

100. D: The educational strategy that is likely to be most effective for a population older than 65 years is audiovisual/print materials because they likely have more experience learning through use of these types of materials. Health fairs, social networking, and role playing are more likely to appeal to a young population, but this generalization may not be true for all individuals. It is important to have a good understanding of the priority population and to gear educational strategies to their preferred learning methods when possible.

101. C: An example of an intervention at the primary level of prevention is conducting stroke-screening tests at local pharmacies, supermarkets, and recreation centers. Primary prevention aims to prevent disease, such as by reducing risk factors and toxic exposures and by identifying people at risk, such as through mass screening programs and immunizations. Secondary prevention takes place after diagnosis and aims to reduce the adverse effects of disease, such as through adequate treatment, routine exams, and modifications in lifestyle. Tertiary prevention aims to assist people with long-term health problems to better manage their disease and improve their quality of life.

102. D: If the health education specialist wants to inform people about classes but the socioeconomic status and cultural backgrounds of the priority populations at three retirement communities are quite different, the best initial step is to convene focus groups to discuss the best methods of communicating to members of the different groups. The health education specialist, for example, may find that radio is commonly listened to in all three communities but newspapers are commonly subscribed to in only one community.

103. A: If an assessment instrument yields consistent test rests in different events (test-retest), then the instrument is said to have reliability. Reliability refers to the scores or results of testing, not to the items on the instrument. Instruments should have enough reliability that the scores derived from testing can be trusted even though 100% reliability is essentially impossible to achieve. Measures of reliability include test-retest, parallel form reliability, internal consistency, and split-half reliability coefficient.

104. C: Informed consent for those participating in research includes the nature/purpose of a project, the risk associated with participation, and the benefits of participation; however, informed consent does not include the penalty for stopping participation in a project because participants must be allowed to stop participation whenever they choose without penalty. If a penalty were to be applied when a participant wanted to stop participation, this would be a form of coercion.

105. B: If a web-based testing instrument assessing knowledge about food and nutrition shows similar results to one-on-one testing, the web-based instrument is said to have criterion-related validity (or instrumental validity). Criterion-related validity results from comparing the scores derived from testing with one instrument (web-based testing) to another that has been previously validated (one-on-one testing). Other types of validity include face validity (appearance of validity), content validity (degree to which it reflects the domain tested), and construct validity (convergent and discriminate).

106. B: If data collection includes four different paper surveys and data must be evaluated on an individual as well as group basis, the best method of data storage is to use color-coded surveys in individual folders, being sure that each survey contains the correct subject code and is placed in the appropriate folder. Color-coding is especially important when the data are evaluated for the group. Even if the information is to be entered into the computer, the original documents should remain in storage.

107. D: If using a commercial survey company to collect and manage electronic data, it is most important for the health education specialist to investigate security because electronic data is at risk of corruption or loss if a server crashes and may also be at risk of hacking. Data should be backed up and encrypted in such a way that confidentiality is protected. Additionally, access should be by authorization only, and strong passwords should be required for access.

108. B: An institutional review board (IRB) must be comprised of at least 5 members from various backgrounds (educational, ethnic, gender, socioeconomic, cultural). If a protected population—pregnant women, children, infants, prisoners, or cognitively impaired individuals—is to be included in the research, then a member of that population or someone with experience working with the population must be included as a member of the IRB. Members must have adequate expertise in reviewing research and must not have a conflict of interest.

109. A: If the health impact assessment (HIA) identifies possible adverse health effects resulting from a proposed project, the next action is to develop recommendations for project changes in order to mitigate the adverse health effects. These recommendations then will be reviewed by the decision makers to determine what, if any, changes should be made to the project. Recommendations should be evidence based and should outline how the changes will reduce risk to the target population.

110. C: If as part of a cancer prevention program, the health education specialist surveys a group of patients with ovarian cancer to determine what lifestyle choices may have led to development of this form of cancer, this type of study is categorized as retrospective. In a retrospective study, the proposed cause (lifestyle choices) and the effect (ovarian cancer) have already taken place. The group, in this case, is referred to as a cohort because the members have the same characteristic (ovarian cancer).

111. D: When providing health education to Native Americans to encourage more use of Western medicine for chronic health problems, such as heart disease and diabetes, the best title for the class is probably, "Combining Western Medicine and Native American Healing." There are over 500 Native American tribes, and there are many differences among them, but traditional practices must be respected. In many cases, patients can benefit from both Western medicine and healers, who can provide much emotional support.

112. C: If, as part of a needs assessment, the health education specialist is considering the use of an internet survey in order to reduce costs, the health education specialist should first consider internet access, including high-speed internet, as well as computer literacy of the priority population. Because participation with online surveys is often low, the health education specialist must also consider methods to increase participation and determine the number of surveys needed to provide an adequate sampling.

113. A: The three most important components of the teaching plan are the purpose, goals, and objectives, because the other components are all in support of these three. The purpose is the reason for the lesson, the goal is the end result that the instructor wants to achieve by the lesson, and the objectives are the measurable achievements that should result from the lesson. The teaching plan should include the method of instruction and the time allotted for each activity as well as the resources needed to complete the lesson and the method of evaluation.

114. B: When developing a health education program for a large priority population, in order to ensure that community feedback is included, the most effective solution for the health education specialist is a community advisory board, which should include a representative cross-section of the population and should meet regularly. The community advisory board may provide not only feedback but also guidance in the form of strategies or interventions that may best meet the needs of the population.

115. D: The Plain Writing Act of 2010, which applies to federal agencies, requires that communications be understandable to the average person. The law applies to written documents as well as text on websites, social media, and all print and electronic materials, including informed consent. Although it does not apply to other agencies, the health education specialist should use plain language, avoiding jargon and excessively technical language, when communicating to priority populations and stakeholders to ensure that the information is interpreted correctly.

116. A: If the health education specialist is unsure about the legal standards that may apply to a project, the best solution for the health education specialist is to consult legal counsel, but the counsel should have experience dealing with legal standards related to the project. Depending on the agency involved in the project and the state in which the project is to be carried out, concerns may include compliance with state and federal regulations, such as ADA compliance and plain language requirements.

117. B: During the *contemplation* stage of change, the health education specialist should support the learner's decision making for change by focusing on benefits of change and methods of dealing with obstacles. The stages of change include:

- Precontemplation: Discuss negative consequences of action in nonjudgmental manner.
- Contemplation: (see above)
- Preparation: Provide guidance on effective methods and positive reinforcement, and help to develop realistic goals.

- Action: Encourage practice with new behavior, provide rewards and incentives, and assist to self-monitor changes.
- Maintenance: Provide encouragement and support.

118. D: In a project that spans a multi-county area with large distances between project members, the best method to use to discuss problems and findings on a weekly basis is probably videoconferencing. Videoconferencing is less time consuming than travel. Being able to hear and see each other facilitates discussion. A number of options are available depending on the number of participants, but costs are relatively low with some versions free, although more sophisticated systems may be costly.

119. B: If the health education specialist convinces a person to participate in a program that will benefit the person but fails to tell the person everything involved in participation because of the fear the person will not agree, the ethical principle that has been breached is autonomy. Withholding the information interfered with the person's right to self-determination—whether it results in making a good or poor decision—because the person was not able to give informed consent with complete information.

120. A: With McKenzie et al's five generic phases of program implementation, once a program has been adopted, the next step is to identify necessary tasks and prioritize them. Then, a system of management must be established and the plans actually put into action. This can be done in a variety of ways, such as through pilot or field testing, phasing in, or total implementation. The last step is to end the program or to take steps to sustain it.

121. A: The best way to assess technology needs for a large-scale multi-level program is to hire a consultant. Investing in the wrong kind or inadequate technology can be a costly mistake in terms of time, money, and implementation. The health education specialist should outline as completely as possible what is expected of the technology in terms of input and output as well as the number of users and the types of access needed. The consultant must also be aware of budget constraints.

122. C: If the health education specialist finds that participants routinely do internet searches about their conditions and question every aspect of a risk-reduction program, wanting to assert some control over their choices, this is an example of *consumer empowerment,* which is a movement toward increasingly asserting autonomy. The internet has allowed people to quickly and easily access information without the aid of health professionals, and as people become better informed, they tend to want more control.

123. A: If a program is using store-and-forward telehealth technology to monitor clinical data (BP, pulse, ECG), the health education specialist expects clinical data to be stored on the device and then transmitted at specified times, often over a telephone or the internet. For example, images, videos, clinical data, and/or audio can be captured by a device and then stored on the device itself or in a computer and then forwarded to a physician or other specialist at a later time for review.

124. B: If when evaluating a partnership, the health education specialist finds that one partner in the agreement had failed to meet its financial obligations because of unexpected loss of a large grant, forcing the other partner to contribute additional funds to carry out the joint program, the best solution at this point is probably to renegotiate the partnership because there may be value to the partnership beyond financial contribution. However, this will depend on the members and their willingness to work together.

125. C: When developing a logic model to serve as a guide for program development, the health education specialist should first describe expected outcomes because it is necessary to know what a program expects to do before the steps to achieving it can be realized. The short-term and long-term outcomes should be outlined first and then the impact of the program (usually in 5-10 years). Once the outcomes are identified, the activities and resources to carry out the activities should be outlined.

126. D: When identifying evidence to justify a public health program, the best database in which to look for public health data is CDC Wonder (wonder.cdc.gov). Wide-ranging Online Data for Epidemiologic Research (WONDER) is a single-point access to retrieve data from various government sources, such as the CDC, NIOSH, NCI, NCEH, and NCCDPHP. The database contains published documents and reports as well as numeric data that can be downloaded into text or spreadsheet programs.

127. B: A PEST analysis looks at the following factors: P) political, (E) economic, (S) social, and (T) technological. The purpose of the PEST analysis is to assess what effects these factors will have on a program. As part of adequate communication, the health education specialist should identify both the positive and negative aspects of each factor, the reasons that the factors will affect the program. and mitigating steps that can be taken to minimize negative effects.

128. A: If the health education specialist has arranged for a nutritionist to give a series of cooking classes throughout a Native American community in order to teach members how to lower the fat content of their familiar foods or to use healthier fats, this is an example of cultural care accommodation. Cultural care accommodation allows people to continue with their cultural practices but attempts to help them modify some aspects so they are more healthful.

129. C: If the health education specialist attends a community meeting and asks a number of key figures as well as members of the general public unstructured questions about community needs, problems, and strengths, this type of assessment is referred to as informant interview. Informant interviews may include random telephone surveys and person-on-the-street interviews. Participant observation involves observation of informal or formal community activities without questioning in order to get an overall impression of needs or concerns.

130. D: If the people in a priority population tend to believe that illness is caused by supernatural influences, such as evil spirits or spells placed on them by others, this health belief system is referred to as *magico-religious*. People with this belief system may seek out spiritualists who can remove evil "spells," at the same time that they participate in Western medical programs and take Western medications, and those who work with people with this belief system must realize that these beliefs are very powerful.

131. D: A program to help children with lead exposure–related developmental delays is an example of a tertiary intervention at the community level of public health practice. Tertiary interventions are those that take place for a group who already have a condition in order to prevent further deterioration and to improve the quality of life. Primary interventions are those aimed to prevent a disease or condition. Secondary interventions focus on reducing the impact of a disease or condition that exists, such as by early diagnosis and treatment.

132. C: Considering the 4 Ps of social marketing, the focus when the health education specialist is considering how information will reach the priority population is *place.* The 4 Ps:

- Product: This may be tangible (such as equipment or goods) or intangible (such as information).
- Price: This is the effort/cost required of the consumer to gain the product.
- Place: This refers to the method of distribution, the way in which the product gets to the consumer.
- Promotion: This is the marketing approach, including the use of media.

133. A: The process that commits two or more persons or organizations to reach a common goal by enhancing the capacity of all or one is collaboration. Collaborations should involve shared goals and shared workload. Collaboration usually requires some type of leadership because collaboration often works best with some structure, although the leadership position may be informal. With a true collaboration, all parties should benefit in some manner. Collaboration software may be used to improve communication among those involved in the collaboration.

134. D: Ratio data includes weight because a finding of zero (0) means the absence of weight, a criterion for ratio data. With ratio data, when the number doubles, the quantity doubles, so 4 is twice as much as 2. Ratio data can be added and subtracted, and mean, median, percentile, standard deviation, and frequency distribution calculated. Height is another example of ratio data, but temperature in Celsius or Fahrenheit is not because a finding of zero (0) does not mean an absence of temperature. However, if using temperature in Kelvin, a finding of zero (0) does mean the absence of all temperature, so Kelvin temperatures are not ratio data.

135. B: If the health education specialist helps family members to understand their feelings about one family member's schizophrenia, this type of intervention is affective because it deals with feelings, beliefs, and values. A cognitive intervention would be to provide the family members factual information about the mental disease. A behavioral intervention would entail teaching the family members how to carry out specific tasks, such as administering medications or taking safety precautions if self-injury or other-directed violence is a concern.

136. A: When using the AIDES method in order to improve medication and treatment adherence in a program to enhance the quality of life for older adults with COPD, the steps include:

- Assess: The current status and desired status should be assessed.
- Individualize: The health education specialist collaborates with the individual to create a plan that fits the needs of that person.
- Document: The plan and interventions are carefully documented in an appropriate manner.
- Educate: The individual is provided the appropriate education to meet his or her needs.
- Supervise: The individual is supervised to ascertain progress.

137. C: If the health education specialist has implemented a program for post-stroke individuals with aphasia, there is no need to speak slowly and deliberately. The speaker should use a normal speaking voice. Other interventions may include the use of assistive devices, such as letter boards, picture boards, or computer programs. It is especially important to be patient and to freely praise and encourage individuals with aphasia because they may become very frustrated when trying to communicate.

138. B: GIS (geographic information system) technology may be the most effective to aid in research regarding the health effects of air pollution on a priority population in a widespread area.

GIS technology can capture geographical data, as well as store, assess, and present the data. GIS mapping can, for example, provide a visual representation of the extent of health effects related to air pollution and can help to identify sources of pollution as well by showing the areas most affected.

139. D: The purpose of a culture audit at an organization is to assess the overall perceptions and values of an organization. The culture audit looks at the culture of the organization at all different levels. Culture audits may include surveys to ascertain how individuals feel about the organization, observations, focus groups, and review of documents. A culture audit should review the power structure of an organization and attitudes toward the power structure as well as the social structure.

140. C: The amount of green space in a community is a physical determinant of health because it is a part of the natural environment, which also includes the weather. Other physical determinants include buildings and infrastructure (such as roads and bridges), housing, design of the community, physical barriers (such as lack of elevators), and physical hazards (such as exposure to toxins). Physical determinants also include aesthetic elements (such as adequate lighting and landscaping).

141. A: If a community health organization replaces the direction and program managers because of a desire to move in a different direction, this approach to change is revolutionary in the sense that the change is abrupt and involves a sudden and perhaps extensive change in the organization. Revolutionary changes can be very disruptive and may face obstruction by those who have not been a party to the change, although the changes may be productive in the long run.

142. D: When considering the need to recruit individuals to fill positions for a program that is in the planning stage, a concern is the reason the position is required because personnel can be a major expense. The consideration should include whether or not a new hire is necessary or an existing employee or volunteer can assume the position. If the position is necessary, then the logistics of recruitment should be considered at a later phase, such as immediately before or during implementation.

143. B: According to the Census Bureau chart for children receiving food stamps (Graph 4), the living situation that has resulted in the greatest increase in the percentage of children in need of nutritional assistance is one with two unmarried parents. While living situations with mother only has the largest overall percentage, the increase from 2007 to 2014 was 14%. With two unmarried parents, the increase from 2007 to 2015 was 17%. This increase may reflect the increasing trend for couples to raise children together without being married.

144. B: According to Graph 4, the living arrangement that resulted in the least change in the percentage of children receiving food stamps is married parents, increasing only 6% (from 5% to 11%). Considering that the greatest increase occurred in a living arrangement with two unmarried parents, this difference probably reflects the fact that people with higher socioeconomic status (who are less likely to need food stamps) tend to marry at higher rates than those with lower socioeconomic status.

145. C: The HaPI (Health and Psychosocial Instruments) database would provide the best resource for a health education specialist who is researching measurement tools and instruments. HaPI covers many types of measurement instruments, including questionnaires, tests, surveys, interviews, and checklists. The database includes journals (peer-reviewed), books, reports, and publisher's catalogs from various professions. The information covers tools and instruments from a variety of fields, including medicine, public health, social work, psychology, human resources, and communication.

146. B: If when trying to replicate an evidence-based program for reduction of teen pregnancy the health education specialist needed to extensively modify some parts of the program in order to meet local policy guidelines and community suitability, he or she must also likely modify the outcomes evaluation. Different procedures and processes are not likely to lead to the same outcomes or even the same methods of assessing outcomes, so the outcomes evaluation must be carefully assessed and modified accordingly.

147. B: If an individual tells the health education specialist that he is considering discontinuing his medications and controlling his diabetes with a high-protein diet based on information he found in a blog post on the internet, the health education specialist should advise the individual to seek information from a valid source, such as a nutritionist, physician, government agency, or organization, such as the American Diabetes Association. The individual should be advised that anyone can say virtually anything online with no evidence required, so information in blogs should be viewed with suspicion.

148. D: If the members of a nonprofit agency that conducts a free health clinic want to access information about recommended immunizations for children and adults, the health education specialist should refer them to the CDC. The CDC provides children and adult immunization schedules, updated annually. Information is provided for consumers and for healthcare professionals. The CDC also provides detailed information about the different vaccines, including any adverse effects that may occur, such as allergic reactions.

149. A: If the health education specialist is doing research to locate charitable organizations that might donate funds for a suicide prevention program that the health education specialist wants to implement, the best online resource is Candid. Candid was created by the merger of the Foundation Center and GuideStar. Candid provides an extensive database of philanthropic organizations and lists thousands of foundations, providing information and links for individual grant seekers and nonprofit grant seekers. Candid also provides a search function so that the grant seeker can immediately access a list of grants available for the topic of interest.

150. A: The best choice for a "safe" change to make when preparing evidence-based guidelines for a priority population is modification of language to reduce medical and technical jargon. Modifications may also be done to account for age, gender, or ethnic background. Removing information or condensing information should be done judiciously as doing so may profoundly alter the intent of the material. Added information should be clearly identified so that it does not appear to be part of the original material, and it should only be added if it is evidence based and validated.

151. B: When determining what method of presentation to use when sharing information about a program, the first consideration is the audience. The health education specialist should consider the knowledge base of the audience, as this will guide how technical the presentation should be. The audience status/position (general public, health professionals, politicians, corporate managers) may also help the health education specialist determine whether a presentation should be formal or informal, and the size of the audience will also determine how the material is presented.

152. D: If a health education specialist who works with four high schools in the county needs to determine what health-related information is most needed by the students, the most efficient method to gain information is surveys. Instructors' opinions may be biased or inaccurate, and interviewing enough randomly chosen students to have a valid sampling can be very time consuming. Because four schools are involved, focus groups may not be effective. Surveys are fairly easy to design and can be easy to assess statistically, depending on how the survey is written.

153. C: If the health education specialist must give a presentation to the board of directors of a sponsoring organization, he or she should plan to give a formal presentation. The health education specialist should dress formally (such as in a suit) and should plan to provide statistics and graphs using projection software (such as slide shows) if possible, during the presentation to better convey information. The level of language should be consistent with the educational background of the members.

154. B: If a client considers different exercise programs and chooses one that provides the most benefit, according to the Elaboration Likelihood Model of communication, this is an example of the process of persuasion by the central route. This theory states that people are persuaded to action by reasoning. Persuasion by the central route involves consideration and analysis of the message in order to make a decision. People can also be persuaded by the peripheral route, which involves less personal involvement and is often influenced by marketing.

155. D: The health education specialist is involved in advocacy when he or she addresses the county board of supervisors about the importance of cleaning up a park. Advocacy requires speaking up and trying to convince others. Participating in cleanup is a service, not advocacy. Voting against politicians who refused to provide funding and believing in the necessity of cleaning up the park are personal actions but do not necessarily influence others to take action.

156. B: The Public Health Accreditation Board (PHAB) is a nonprofit accreditation agency for public health services, including tribal, state, local and territorial. PHAB provides standards and measures to help departments prepare for accreditation and education services to help with technical issues, guidance, online orientation, a guide for accreditation, newsletters, and videos. Participation in PHAB's accreditation program is voluntary with fees for participation based on the size of the population served by the health department.

157. D: Resource materials obtained from an online site should be evaluated for:

- Accuracy: Determine how the site is funded and by whom, the purpose of the site, and the credentials of those involved in order to determine whether the information is reliable.
- Relevance: Evaluate whether the material addresses the needs and contains information that is helpful and useful.
- Timeliness: Check to ensure that the material is up-to-date and has not been superseded by newer information.

158. A: If a client is able to read and understand a consent form, according to the National Adult Literacy Survey categorizations, the person is said to have literacy related to document tasks, which are also involved in the ability to read insurance reports and bus or train schedules. Another type of literacy task is prose tasks, which involve reading with comprehension and the ability to understand the themes found in poetry, books, magazines, and journals. Quantitative tasks involve working with numbers embedded in written material, such as understanding prices on a menu or bill, figuring out taxes, or calculating the number of carbohydrates consumed.

159. B: While all of these (costs, instructing clients, rules of use) are important, the primary concern with including a message board as part of a website is the need to monitor the website. If the message board is open to everyone, there is a risk that trolls (people who purposely write negative comments to cause discontent) will invade the site. Even if the message board requires membership and passwords, people can become verbally abusive to others. The health education specialist must plan for monitoring, but this can be expensive and/or time consuming.

160. C: When planning a media campaign to promote a program, television is likely to have the largest audience reach. The ability to combine visual and audio elements facilitates emotional appeals or demonstrations. Even low-income and low-literacy audiences are more likely to watch television than to access other media. However, paid ads tend to be expensive, and public service announcements often run at times when few are watching TV. Also, if the audience is large and the program small, the response may exceed the program's abilities.

161. B: When conducting community-based teaching with older adults, it is best to limit sessions to 20-30 minutes. If a longer time is needed, then a 10- to 15-minute break should be provided to allow participants to move about, relax, or take a restroom break. If possible, the room should be quiet and well lit, and the health education specialist should face the participants and speak in a slow, clear voice to help facilitate lip reading for those with hearing impairments. Written materials should use a large font size.

162. A: The five elements of an advocacy plan are as follows: 1) goals, (2) organizational considerations, (3) constituents, allies, and opponents, (4) targets, and (5) tactics. The last element (tactics) is critical because these involve the actions that will be carried out in order to meet the goals. The health education specialist must carefully assess the various communication channels and communication strategies in determining what type of tactics to use to gain the necessary support.

163. D: When selecting an instrument for data collection, the first question to ask is, "Does the instrument measure the correct data?" If it does not, then it is not appropriate. Choosing the correct instrument is critical to the success of data collection, so the instrument should be considered carefully to ensure it is well written and constructed. The instrument should measure the intended variables and should be sensitive to small differences. Other issues to consider are ease of administration, readability, and costs.

164. B: If the object of data collection is to assess patterns of discharge from a healthcare facility, the best initial method is probably record review. The discharge summary should contain most of the necessary data, including the length of stay, the diagnosis, the discharge plan, and the place to which the person is discharged. Additionally, the discharge plan should list medications, follow-up treatment, and appointments. If the purpose of data collection is to determine the efficacy of the discharge procedures, then surveys and interviews may be indicated.

165. B: Facebook, LinkedIn, Twitter, and SnapChat are examples of social media. Social media is increasingly used for marketing, especially to younger generations who are familiar with computers and the internet. Content developed for social media should be highly focused and of good quality if it is to attract an audience. Taking the time to identify and target influential individuals is an essential strategy in marketing because they can share content and expand outreach at no additional cost.

Practice Test #2

1. The health education specialist must work with the IT consultant to ensure that the information system used for a health promotion program protects both the data and system. An inherent weakness in a system design resulting from inadequate risk management and testing is categorized as a(n):

a. threat.
b. vulnerability.
c. attack.
d. deficit.

2. Kirkpatrick's four-level training evaluation method comprises the levels of:

a. input, manipulation, output, and outcomes.
b. question, view, monitor, and evaluate.
c. reason, learn, monitor, and assess.
d. reaction, learning, behavior, and results.

3. When the health education specialist is assessing the need for health-related information, the initial step is to:

a. identify the needs.
b. organize materials.
c. match need to source material.
d. assess the quality of materials.

4. According to the American School Health Association, all of the following are aspects of school health except:

a. nutritious foods.
b. advanced placement classes.
c. programs of physical activity.
d. health education.

5. If the health education specialist chooses a software option for instructional purposes that is the easiest for participants to use but the most difficult for educators because of a complex interface for entering content, the health education specialist is applying the ethical principle of:

a. equity.
b. beneficence.
c. autonomy.
d. non-maleficence.

6. According to the principle standard of the *National Standards for Culturally and Linguistically Appropriate Services in Health and Health Care*, health care providers should be respectful of and responsive to "diverse cultural health beliefs and practices, preferred languages, health literacy and:

a. individual needs."
b. socioeconomic status."
c. conflicts and complaints."
d. other communication needs."

7. If collaboration among a priority population, partners, and other stakeholders is important for success of an education program, the health education specialist should:

a. explain the importance of collaboration.
b. outline the steps in collaboration.
c. elicit input during planning.
d. elicit responses to the plan before implementation.

8. When considering the impact of delivered messages to a priority population, *reach* refers to:

a. the number of individuals who see/hear the message.
b. the area in which the message is broadcast.
c. how well individuals recall hearing/seeing the message.
d. the costs entailed in producing the message.

9. An example of a primary prevention study is:

a. review of 5 years of demographic data regarding rates of influenza.
b. assessing rates of influenza in two different age groups.
c. assessing rates of influenza prior to implementation of a campaign to increase immunizations.
d. assessing decreased rates of influenza after a campaign to increase immunizations.

10. The primary focus of the Elaboration Likelihood Model of communication is:

a. persuasion.
b. avoidance of tension.
c. compromise.
d. dominance.

11. When using an interpreter to communicate with a non-English speaker, the health education specialist should do all of the following except:

a. use an interpreter of the same gender.
b. direct statements and questions to the interpreter.
c. speak in a normal tone of voice.
d. use a qualified professional interpreter.

12. According to the *Federal Plain Language Guidelines*, which of the following sentences would be preferred in documents intended for the priority population?

a. "The information is for the reader's use."
b. "The information is for our use."
c. "The information is for your use."
d. "The information is for his/her use."

13. With the MATCH planning model, the primary task to complete during the first phase is:

a. planning interventions.
b. preparing for implementation.
c. evaluating.
d. selecting goals.

14. If a needs assessment shows that one community offers more services to older adults than those offered in another community, the type of need this represents is:

a. relative.
b. normative.
c. perceived.
d. expressed.

15. According to the CDC's workplace health promotion, when implementing an organizational program to increase breast cancer screening, the best approach to increase mammography screening is:

a. videos.
b. pamphlets/posters.
c. survey.
d. one-on-one education.

16. If, during data collection, serendipitous findings emerge, the best approach is to:

a. ignore the findings.
b. modify the project.
c. record findings for future research.
d. redirect the research toward the serendipitous findings.

17. The maximum number of words per slide when using projection software, such as PowerPoint, should be:

a. 25.
b. 50.
c. 75.
d. 100.

18. A health education specialist who is working with a predominately Muslim population must set up a series of appointments with individuals. The appointments are specifically scheduled between prayer times so that they do not interfere with the individuals' religious practice. This is an example of:

a. cultural care preservation.
b. cultural care accommodation.
c. cultural care restructuring.
d. cultural care capitulation.

19. A professional development plan could include all of the following except:

a. reading professional journal articles about health education.
b. authoring a journal article about health education.
c. reading about health education needs in the popular press.
d. making a conference presentation about health education.

20. Which Boolean operator should be used most sparingly?

a. NEAR
b. NOT
c. AND
d. OR

Questions 21-23 refer to the following information:

Graph 1

Gonorrhea - Rates of Reported Cases Among Woman Aged 15-24 Years of Age by State, United States and Outlying Areas, 2022

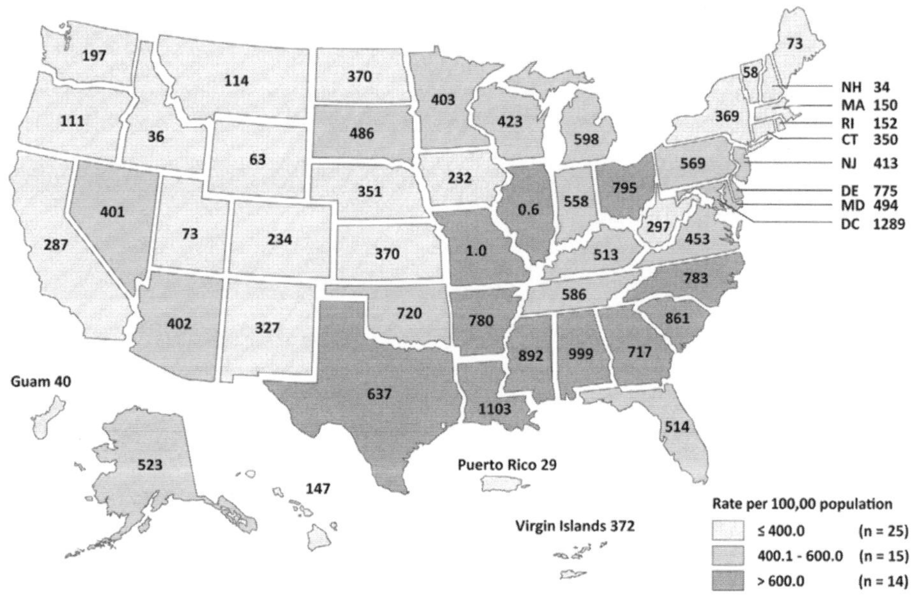

21. Based on the Graph 1, which area of the United States has the highest rate of gonorrhea among women aged 15-24?

a. Northeast
b. Northwest
c. Southwest
d. Southeast

22. If utilizing the data in Graph 1 as part of planning, this type of data would be considered secondary, which is classified according to:

a. the type of data.
b. the entity that collected the data.
c. the time period in which the data was collected.
d. the ability to quantify the data.

23. According to Graph 1, the health education specialist can conclude that the Northwest:

a. has the lowest rates of gonorrhea.
b. has lower rates because of low population.
c. contains the state with the lowest rate of gonorrhea.
d. has better sex education than other states.

24. When conducting qualitative research, the literature review may be deferred until after all data are collected:

a. because a literature review is not needed.
b. because this is standard protocol.
c. to save time at the onset of the project.
d. to avoid the review influencing the research.

25. The HIPAA privacy rule protects:

a. individually identifiable health information.
b. research institutions.
c. individual researchers.
d. electronic information.

26. A culture audit most often begins with:

a. observations.
b. surveys.
c. consultant reports.
d. complaints.

27. Which of the following is an indication of ethical rigor when determining the validity of qualitative research?

a. research reveals identity of participants
b. participants were unaware of the research
c. consent was obtained and documented
d. participants were rewarded for inclusion in research

28. When determining the time frame needed to collect data, the best solution may be to:

a. conduct a pilot study.
b. use an existing model.
c. double the estimated time.
d. estimate based on best guess.

29. The first task in data collection is:

a. collecting data systematically.
b. selecting subjects.
c. maintaining research controls.
d. solving problems.

30. An example of a potential research subject who would most likely be classified as having *diminished autonomy* is:

a. a person with an above the knee amputation.
b. a non-English speaker.
c. a person older than 65 years.
d. a person with bipolar disorder.

31. The best method to follow in order to plan for technical failure is to:

a. routinely back up files.
b. properly maintain equipment.
c. store only to portable memory devices.
d. learn to troubleshoot equipment.

32. The first step in obtaining an appropriate data collection instrument for a large-scale study is to:

a. design a data collection instrument.
b. ask fellow researchers for recommendations.
c. conduct a literature review.
d. modify instruments used for other research.

33. When collecting data about rates of influenza, a good source of secondary data is:

a. CDC.
b. CMS.
c. SAMSHA.
d. FDA.

34. If a needs assessment determines whether children in the community are immunized against whooping cough, the type of need this focuses on is:

a. expressed.
b. normative.
c. perceived.
d. comparative.

35. If the health education specialist wants to measure the self-confidence of adolescents participating in a risk-reduction program, in order to have content validity, the health education specialist must first:

a. find a comparison instrument.
b. develop questions.
c. form a focus group.
d. define the domain.

36. With the PRECEDE-PROCEED model for planning in health education, the last phase of PROCEED involves:

a. process evaluation.
b. administrative/policy assessment.
c. outcomes evaluation.
d. impact evaluation.

37. Which of the following modifications in behavior is likely to have the most impact on health?

a. utilization of public transportation
b. smoking cessation
c. use of medical marijuana
d. change to a vegetarian diet

38. The purpose of receiving the CHES certification is to:

a. demonstrate mastery of necessary skills across all practice areas.
b. demonstrate mastery of necessary skills in one practice area.
c. demonstrate motivation to succeed in the field.
d. meet state requirements for employment.

Questions 39-42 refer to the following information:

Scenario A

A community with a low-income population is faced with high rates of adolescent pregnancy resulting in increased high school dropout rates as well as increased utilization of well-baby clinics and the WIC program, and enrollment in public assistance programs. In consultation with the local health department, the health education specialist is going to plan a program to decrease the rate of pregnancy among adolescents.

39. The health education specialist begins to gather information about the priority population by conducting a needs assessment. When conducting a needs assessment utilizing the three-phase model (explore, gather/analyze data, and make decisions), the first phase includes:

a. setting priority needs.
b. determining the target population.
c. identifying areas of concern.
d. gathering data.

40. The health education specialist identifies a number of different needs and possible interventions, but funds are limited, so the interventions must be prioritized. When utilizing a strategy grid to prioritize, and *need* and *cost* are the criteria selected, which of the following categories probably has the highest priority?

a. low need/high cost
b. low need/low cost
c. high need/high cost
d. high need/low cost

41. If, as one of the interventions to reduce pregnancy rates, the health education specialist plans a high school education program to prevent pregnancy in collaboration with the school district, the most critical element to consider is:

a. policy.
b. financial support.
c. religion.
d. culture.

42. If a number of key individuals in the community have been vociferous in their disapproval of a program because they fear it will encourage promiscuity and have influenced others to oppose the program, which communication theory does this exemplify?

a. attribution
b. cognitive dissonance
c. contagion
d. knowledge gap.

43. The primary goal of the Directors of Health Promotion and Education (DHPE) is:

a. prevention.
b. health equity.
c. rehabilitation.
d. education.

44. Which of the following factors has the most impact on health behaviors?

a. religion
b. place of residence
c. race
d. socioeconomic status

45. If the trend toward increased use of e-cigarettes continues, the impact on health is likely to be:

a. positive.
b. negative.
c. both negative and positive.
d. negligible.

46. When attempting to engage a priority population in participating in assessment, the best method is likely to:

a. show how participants benefit.
b. pay people to participate.
c. appeal to social consciousness.
d. apply punitive measures for non-participation.

47. A mission statement generally reflects:

a. past achievements.
b. future goals.
c. current status
d. financial resources.

48. When preparing a visual display showing the results of a needs assessment for a presentation to community representatives, the best method of display is usually a:

a. histogram.
b. line graph.
c. pie chart.
d. bar graph.

49. Which of the following databases is likely to provide the best information about school health and school-aged children?

a. ERIC
b. MEDLINE
c. CINAHL
d. EBMR

50. The three domains of learning are:

a. hearing, seeing, and feeling.
b. memorization, utilization, and internalization.
c. cognitive, affective, and psychomotor.
d. acquisition, utilization, and storage.

51. When considering the frame of mind of participants in an educational program in relation to readiness to learn, frame of mind usually involves concern with the:

a. present.
b. past.
c. future needs.
d. future desires.

52. If the goal of data collection is to assess participant satisfaction with education provided in a community-wide program, the best initial method is probably:

a. interviews.
b. focus groups.
c. surveys.
d. records review.

53. Which of the following is an example of a well-written objective?

a. "Participants will be able to describe the health risks of smoking."
b. "Following a class on smoking cessation, the participants will be able to understand the health risks of smoking."
c. "Following a class on smoking cessation, the participants will agree to stop smoking."
d. "Following a class on smoking cessation, the participants will be able to list 4 health risks associated with smoking."

Questions 54 and 55 refer to the following information:

Graph 2

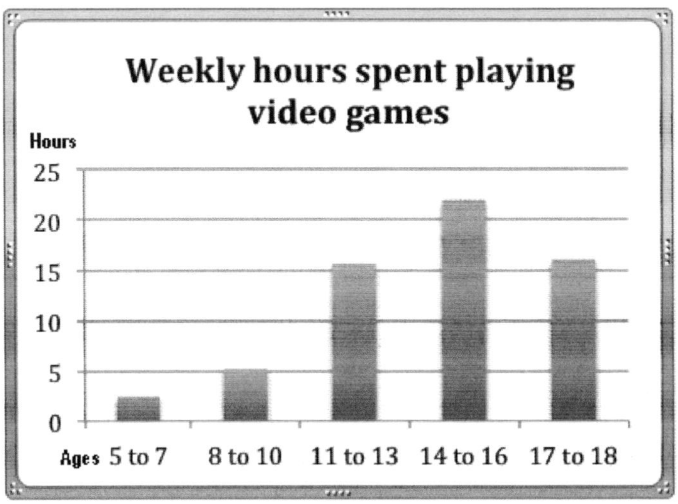

54. The health education specialist conducted school surveys to determine how many average hours students spent playing video games per week. Based on Graph 2, the greatest change in weekly hours playing video games occurred between ages:

a. 7 and 8.
b. 10 and 11.
c. 13 and 14.
d. 16 and 17.

55. Considering the results of the survey illustrated in Graph 2 above, if planning an educational program to highlight the importance of decreasing hours of video game playing, which group should be the priority population to whom the program is directed?

a. preadolescents
b. adolescents
c. teachers
d. parents

56. Physical readiness to learn is most affected by:

a. learning style.
b. cultural background.
c. cognitive ability.
d. task complexity.

57. According to Healthy People 2030, which of the following is considered a social determinant of health?

a. weather
b. physical hazards
c. transportation options
d. work sites

58. The focus of a goal statement should be on:

a. feasibility.
b. current practice.
c. process.
d. end results.

59. When preparing written materials regarding health matters for a community group, at about what grade level should the materials generally be written for?

a. third
b. fifth
c. eighth
d. tenth

60. If designing an educational program about mental health issues for Middle Eastern immigrants, the best course title is probably:

a. Steps to Better Health.
b. Resources for Mental Health Problems.
c. Depression and Other Mental Health Issues.
d. Relieving Emotional Stress.

61. Which of the following is an example of a geographic factor to consider when identifying a priority population?

a. ethnicity
b. gender
c. community
d. workplace

62. The ethical principle that is applied when the health education specialist encourages members of the priority population to help determine the type of educational program that they need is:

a. veracity.
b. beneficence.
c. non-malfeasance.
d. autonomy.

63. If the health education specialist focuses on building relationships within the community and establishing collaboration and power sharing among agencies, the type of leadership the health education specialist is exhibiting is:

a. organizational.
b. strategic.
c. transactional.
d. transformational

64. If an educational program about diabetic prevention targeting Mexican immigrant farmworker families has been meeting at the public health offices but participation has been very low, the best place to consider moving the classes is to:

a. community college in the community.
b. churches in the community.
c. community center.
d. employment office.

65. If the health education specialist has planned a group activity for a class period but participants refuse to cooperate, the best response is to:

a. explain again what is expected.
b. advise participants that cooperation is important.
c. try a different approach.
d. cancel the class.

66. Which of the following sounds is likely to have the most negative effect on learning?

a. intermittent noise from nearby construction
b. steady hum of the air conditioning unit
c. background classical music
d. traffic sounds from nearby freeway

67. In order to be ADA compliant when planning a program, plans must be made to accommodate all of the following except:

a. service animals.
b. personal aides.
c. wheelchairs.
d. comfort animals.

68. When preparing a media bite as part of a campaign of media advocacy to promote an educational program, how long should be media bite be?

a. 5-7 seconds
b. 7-15 seconds
c. 15-30 seconds
d. 3-45 seconds

69. With the CDCynergy model of program planning, before developing communication strategies, it is necessary to:

a. identify/profile the priority population.
b. develop a plan for population evaluation.
c. carry out program development.
d. evaluate available resources.

70. Qualitative methods of assessment are usually part of:

a. summative evaluation.
b. quantitative evaluation.
c. formative evaluation
d. targeted evaluation.

Questions 71-74 refer to the following information:

Scenario B

An inner city has had markedly increased rates of homeless veterans, many with severe mental and substance abuse disorders, resulting in increased citizen complaints and arrests. The health education specialist is planning a multi-level program with the public health department, housing authorities, mental health professionals, and drug rehabilitation centers to reduce homelessness among veterans and to assist them in entering treatment.

71. When eliciting input for the health education plan targeting homeless veterans in the inner city, which of the following organizations may be most helpful?

a. Wounded Warriors
b. Department of Veterans Affairs
c. Veterans of Foreign Wars of the US (VFW)
d. Salvation Army

72. The most important factor in facilitating collaboration efforts among priority population, partners, and other stakeholders is:

a. explaining potential benefits of collaboration.
b. asking for collaboration.
c. outlining problems related to lack of collaboration.
d. demonstrating areas of shared concern.

73. If collecting baseline data to determine the impact of heroin use in the target homeless population, the health education specialist will most likely need to:

a. conduct secondary data collection.
b. conduct primary data collection.
c. conduct a literature review.
d. make observations in the community.

74. A group of community members opposes programs to help homeless veterans because the members believe that the veterans are just looking for a handout because they do not want to work. As an advocate, the best response is to:

a. repudiate the group's claims.
b. challenge the group to provide evidence.
c. reframe the issue.
d. ignore the group.

75. When creating SMART objectives, SMART stands for (1) specific, (2) measurable, (3) attainable, (4) relevant, and (5):

a. tactical.
b. technical.
c. translatable.
d. timely/time-bound.

76. Which learning method is likely to result in the greatest retention?

a. practicing/restating
b. reading
c. listening
d. seeing

77. When using a logic model to plan an education program, which of the following would be categorized as a short-term outcome?

a. decreased rate of smoking among participants after 6 months
b. participants' ability to list adverse effects of nicotine
c. decreased rate of COPD/lung cancer after 20 years
d. decreased incidence of bronchitis and cough

78. The best way to integrate health teaching into a drop-in clinic where large numbers of patients often experience extended waiting periods is by providing:

a. educational posters.
b. informational pamphlets.
c. video presentations.
d. audio recordings.

79. All of the following factors are likely to hinder implementation of an educational program except:

a. media attention.
b. lack of community support.
c. inadequate funding.
d. health education specialist with multiple projects.

80. The health education specialist has developed an educational program that will be implemented by staff members and volunteers at a service agency. Who has the responsibility to ensure that ethical principles are applied to the implementation process?

a. health education specialist
b. staff members
c. volunteers
d. everyone involved in implementation

81. If an education program is to be implemented as part of a research study, the participants:

a. should be verbally informed.
b. should sign informed consent documents.
c. need not be advised about the research.
d. should receive a written explanation of the research.

82. Prior to the first phase of implementation of a new program, a review of the budget shows that the funds for implementation are insufficient, and no further sources of funds can be identified. The best solution is to:

a. discontinue the program.
b. delay implementation in hopes of finding funds.
c. scale back the program.
d. seek to replace paid staff with volunteers.

83. When the health education specialist is recruiting individuals needed for implementation of an education plan, the primary concern is:

a. skills match those needed.
b. good communication skills.
c. physical and emotional health.
d. relationship to priority population.

84. Which of the following is a self-sustaining source of funding for securing resources needed to implement an education plan?

a. application for state grant money
b. receipt of a private donation
c. creation of a nonprofit organization
d. application for grant money from a private company

85. If researching the efficacy of the different types of teaching approaches for a health education program, which database may provide the health education specialist access to the most applicable information?

a. HEDIR
b. ScienceDirect
c. ERIC
d. Google Scholar

86. A survey asks the following question:

How did you hear about this program?
I. newspaper
II. television
III. fliers

This question would be classified as:

a. not mutually exclusive but collectively exhaustive
b. mutually exclusive and collectively exhaustive
c. not mutually exclusive and not collectively exhaustive
d. mutually exclusive but not collectively exhaustive

Questions 87 and 88 refer to the following information:

Graph 3

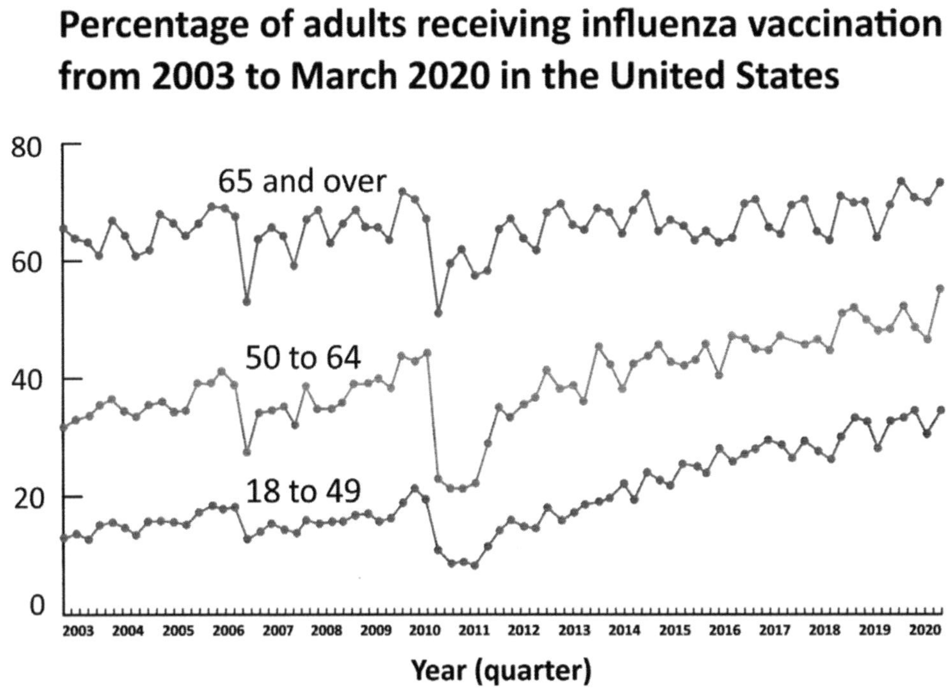

87. Based on Graph 3 showing the percentage of adults in the United States receiving influenza vaccinations, which age group has shown the least improvement in rates since 1997?

a. 65 and older
b. 50-64
c. 18-49
d. data inconclusive

88. If using the data in Graph 3 to determine the priority population to target for education about influenza vaccinations, the education is likely to provide the best long-term outcomes if targeted to which group?

a. 65 and older
b. 50-64
c. 18-49
d. benefit essentially equal for all groups

89. If the health education specialist is creating a Gantt chart as a tool for time and project management, the first step is to:

a. create a project plan identifying tasks and order of completion.
b. create a list of responsible parties for each stage of the project.
c. determine the time frame for the X axis.
d. determine the costs for each activity that will be included.

90. A pilot study showed that even though participants resisted the method of instruction and complained, the health education specialist persisted in using the same method, assuming the participants would later see the value of the method. This could be considered a(n):

a. abuse of authority.
b. good teaching strategy.
c. barrier to learning.
d. enhancement to learning.

91. As part of a marketing plan for a health education program, informational literature is sent out to community members who had previously attended health education classes. This is an example of a:

a. tailored message.
b. targeted message.
c. spam message.
d. random message.

92. If a state has limited Medicaid expansion, leaving many low-income citizens without insurance or access to medical care, this is an example of a:

a. health capacity.
b. political inequity.
c. political capacity.
d. health determinant.

93. If assessing reactions of the participants to a training session in order to modify the course as needed, quantifiable results may best be obtained with:

a. Likert scale.
b. open-ended questions.
c. interviews.
d. yes/no questions.

94. A focus group of inner-city adolescents in a drug treatment program answered questions about drug use. Based on the results of this focus group, a health education plan is to be developed for the county, including a large rural area. Which of the following is the greatest concern?

a. validity
b. reliability
c. generalizability
d. usability

95. A health education specialist is developing a web-based interactive educational program for a federal agency. Section 508 (technical standards) of the Rehabilitation Act requires that the website:

a. involves no cost to the consumer.
b. has text/audio descriptions of any visual displays.
c. uses no visual displays.
d. uses only government-approved software.

96. If the health education specialist at a community hospital is utilizing SWOT analysis to review an educational program about heart health for a primarily low-income population and finds that the community location where the classes are held is no longer on the public transportation bus route, this information would be classified as a(n):

a. strength.
b. weakness.
c. opportunity.
d. threat.

97. The health education specialist is planning advocacy intervention as part of a public health program to reduce the rates of obesity in children and adolescents. Which of the following is an example of advocacy intervention at the systems level?

a. working with school principals to eliminate soft drinks from vending machines
b. asking the board of education to improve the school lunch program
c. meeting with families to discuss their children's activities
d. meeting with children to discuss the need for exercise

98. A health education specialist has devised a number of interventions to increase utilization of a well-baby clinic. These interventions are to be carried out by public health staff. In order to ensure intervention fidelity, an essential element in the program is:

a. training.
b. motivation.
c. supervision.
d. reward.

Questions 99 and 100 refer to the following information:

Scenario C

Most individuals enrolled in a program to decrease the adverse effects associated with hypertension have electronic monitoring devices that transmit daily data that include blood pressure and pulse. This data can be accessed in list form and displayed in line graphs over the internet from secure servers by the project managers as well as the participants.

99. This type of data is referred to as:

a. random data.
b. trend data.
c. snapshot data.
d. individual data.

100. If the electronic monitoring devices are only available to participants who can afford to purchase them and manual recordings must be made by other participants, the ethical principle that has been breached is:

a. equity.
b. beneficence.
c. fidelity.
d. nonmaleficence.

101. If the education plan called for computers and computer-assisted instructional modules to be placed in recreational centers of retirement communities, but data show little use of the equipment, the best solution is to:

a. discontinue the program.
b. provide printed directions.
c. provide a telephone helpline.
d. hold orientation classes.

102. If the health education specialist is advocating for a program to reduce obesity in children and adolescents and believes that billboards for high-sugar soft drinks in the area are targeting minority children, the first step is to:

a. confront the company that owns the billboards.
b. ask the soft drink companies to withdraw the ads.
c. survey all billboards to gather evidence.
d. complain to city management.

103. If gap analysis is being used as part of capacity assessment, the focus is on identifying:

a. current status.
b. deficiencies.
c. successes.
d. future status.

104. A number of activities have been identified as part of development of a Critical Path Method (CPM) work plan. The next step is to:

a. assign times to each activity.
b. identify the resources needed for each activity.
c. identify predecessors and successors.
d. identify input and output.

105. A health education specialist has been depending on low-fidelity simulations for class activities but feels that high-fidelity simulations are necessary for some aspects of training. Which of the following is an example of a high-fidelity simulation?

a. printed posters
b. audiotapes
c. verbal explanation
d. blood pressure cuff

106. As part of a health education program, the health education specialist must teach staff members to master a number of tasks related to phasing in of new medical equipment. The best method to employ is:

a. overview of entire process.
b. low-fidelity simulations.
c. just-in-time presentations.
d. video presentations.

107. When collaborating with others in the development of an education program, the health education specialist presents a potential decision about the project and then makes a final decision based on input from other members of the team. What type of leadership style does this exemplify?

a. participatory
b. democratic
c. consultative
d. bureaucratic

108. Analyzing large amounts of data in order to identify underlying patterns is referred to as:

a. data representation.
b. data mining.
c. data aggregation.
d. data decoding.

109. If a health education specialist is monitoring national rates of rehospitalization of psychiatric patients and comparing them with the internal rates of an institution, this is an example of:

a. internal trending.
b. external benchmarking.
c. data mining.
d. evidence-based practice.

110. If a community agency writes an article about an educational program for free in its print and digital newsletter even though the program is not affiliated with the agency, this is an example of:

a. owned media.
b. paid media.
c. social media.
d. earned media.

111. If the health education specialist is developing a memorandum of understanding (MoU) with another agency in order to implement a joint project, the most important thing to remember about an MoU is that it is a(n):

a. legal contract.
b. informal agreement.
c. record of intent.
d. consulting agreement.

112. When choosing strategies for program implementation, the health education specialist should review the literature to ensure that each strategy has:

a. cost-effectiveness.
b. efficacy.
c. timeliness.
d. efficiency.

113. Which of the following is an example of a workplace implementation of an intervention at the individual level?

a. financial bonus for not smoking
b. smoking cessation program
c. improved lighting and sound reduction
d. development of a mentoring program

114. According to the CDC's Steps to Wellness, the first step to implementing a comprehensive wellness program focusing on physical activity in a workplace is to:

a. plan and assess.
b. promote the plan
c. build support.
d. implement the plan.

115. Which of the following is most likely to be an effective adjunct to a program to prevent, identify, and treat depression?

a. financial advice program
b. environmental safety program
c. substance abuse program
d. physical activity program

116. When analyzing data, which of the following can be computed with nominal data?

a. percentile
b. frequency distribution
c. addition and subtraction
d. mean and median

Questions 117 refers to the following information:

Graph 4

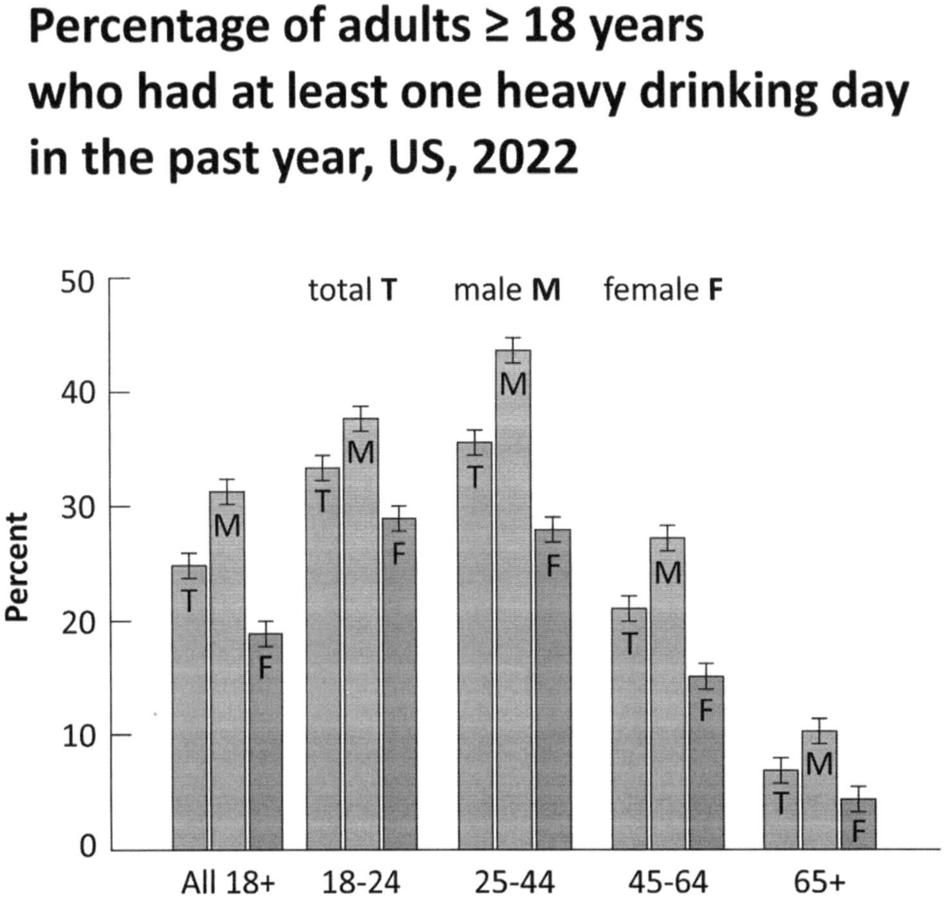

117. According to Graph 4, in which age group is the heavy drinking difference between males and females the least?

a. 18-24
b. 25-44
c. 46-64
d. 65+

118. Assessing outcomes to determine whether they were intended or not is part of:

a. impact evaluation.
b. formative evaluation.
c. summative evaluation.
d. effectiveness evaluation.

119. When selecting items from an existing instrument, the most important factor to consider is:

a. reliability.
b. homogeneity.
c. validity.
d. reproducibility.

120. If an existing instrument includes the item "How frequently do you use communication media (telephone, telegram, FAX) to communicate with friends and family?" which of the following would be an appropriate modification?

a. "How frequently do you use communication media to communicate with others?"
b. "How frequently do you use communication media (telephone, Facebook, Twitter, Instagram, instant messaging, Skype/FaceTime) to communicate with friends and family?"
c. "What types of communication media do you use to communicate with family and friends?"
d. "How frequently do you use social media (Facetime, Instagram, Twitter) to communicate with others?"

121. When data from surveys are to be entered into the computer, the health education specialist must first:

a. check data and resolve problems.
b. ensure data is entered exactly as recorded.
c. determine storage space for data.
d. check power supply to computer.

122. When considering different methods of collecting survey data, the health education specialist recognizes that the benefits of emailed online surveys include all of the following except:

a. lower risk of error.
b. cost-effectiveness.
c. convenience.
d. high rates of response.

123. The purpose of establishing an institutional review board (IRB) in research involving human subjects is:

a. outcomes evaluation.
b. oversight/monitoring.
c. financial guidance.
d. instrument selection.

124. The section of a research report that usually contains descriptions that include words, numbers, and statistics is the:

a. introduction.
b. summary.
c. results.
d. methodology.

125. When considering carrying out a health impact assessment, the initial action should be:

a. scoping.
b. screening.
c. decision making.
d. monitoring.

126. The Framingham study in which a group of participants were monitored for a period of 20 years with a number of different variables assessed is categorized as a:

a. longitudinal study.
b. cross-sectional study.
c. retrospective study.
d. prospective study.

127. All of the following are part of Frieden's 6 components for effective public health program implementation except:

a. utilize innovation for development of the evidence base.
b. utilize both partnerships and coalitions.
c. obtain the necessary resources and support.
d. utilize a large number of high-priority evidence-based interventions.

128. According to the 5 steps involved in the RE-AIM framework from translating research into intervention, the first step (R) refers to:

a. report steps to implementation.
b. recognize various resources.
c. reach the target population.
d. revise initial plans.

129. A public health program to promote maternal and child health focuses on the various factors that affect health, including interpersonal, individual, socioeconomic, institutional, and policy. This is an example of what type of framework?

a. ecological framework (EF)
b. ecosystems service (ES)
c. human-environmental system (HES)
d. the natural step (TNS)

130. If a health education specialist is active in a national organization that aims to improve the health of all Americans by increasing access to care, the focus is on:

a. health equality.
b. health promotion.
c. health disparity.
d. health equity.

131. If a software program has been installed on computers used in an organization in order to monitor who is using the network and the files that are accessed, this type of security tool is a(n):

a. firewall.
b. antivirus program.
c. intrusion detection system.
d. proxy server.

132. Which of the following is the least effective method of communicating an advocacy position to a member of Congress?

a. Email
b. FAX
c. Telephone
d. Mailed latter

133. Historically, when did health education evolve as a true profession?

a. 1940s
b. 1950s
c. 1960s
d. 1970s

134. Which of the following technology options allows people who are collaborating on a project to share, collaborate, and synchronize documents over the internet?

a. Skype
b. Instagram
c. FaceTime
d. Dropbox

135. If the health education specialist sees a need in a program but does not have the financial resources to provide for the need, the best initial approach is to:

a. conduct fundraising events.
b. explore grant opportunities.
c. ask community members for donations.
d. cut costs in other parts of the program.

136. If the health education specialist is recruiting individuals for implementation of a program, which of the following is an acceptable question to ask during the interview?

a. "Do you have any disabilities?"
b. "How old are you?"
c. "Is English your first language?"
d. "Why do you want this position?"

137. The health education specialist must implement a program that will provide educational services to a primarily English-speaking group, but a small subgroup in one community comprises Mexican immigrants with no or little English skills. The best approach is to:

a. provide materials in English.
b. provide materials in English and Spanish.
c. provide a telephone number for Spanish speakers to call for information.
d. provide Spanish-speaking community workers to assist Spanish speakers.

138. As part of program implementation, the electrical wiring must be modified in order to accommodate new technology needs. The most important criterion when selecting a person to do the work is:

a. licensure/certification.
b. experience.
c. recommendations.
d. availability.

139. The health education specialist has facilitated a partnership between two organizations and wants to ensure that the partnership will be effective. Before the partnership is established, the health education specialist should:

a. ask for assurances from the partners.
b. carefully review the partnership agreement.
c. establish an evaluation plan.
d. hire a consultant to review the partnership agreement.

140. When reviewing evidence to justify implementation of a program, the best source for systematic reviews is the:

a. National Library of Medicine.
b. AHRQ.
c. CDC Wonder Online Database.
d. Cochrane Library.

141. When conducting a preliminary assessment of a community, the health education specialist drives through the community and observes the people (race, genders, dress, activities) and the places (boundaries, environment, buildings, housing). This type of assessment is referred to as:

a. drive-by assessment.
b. windshield survey.
c. superficial survey.
d. subjective assessment.

142. The health education specialist is working in a low-income community program with predominately Chinese women to improve the health of mothers and babies, but the health education specialist finds that many mothers stay essentially bedridden for extended periods after giving birth and refuse to bathe or eat or drink cold foods. These practices are based on the health belief system referred to as:

a. humoral.
b. magicoreligious.
c. biomedical.
d. superstition.

143. Population-based public health practice focuses on:

a. an entire population within a community.
b. organization, policies, laws, and power structures.
c. interventions at all levels.
d. attitudes, beliefs, and practices of individuals.

144. According to the attribution model of communication, which of the following is an example of internal attribution?

a. An individual has lost no weight on a weight-loss program and blames the time required to participate.
b. An individual has lost 10 pounds and believes it is because she stayed on a diet and exercised.
c. An individual fails to stay on a diet and blames his spouse for causing him to fail.
d. An individual joins an exercise program with a friend but quits when the friend does.

145. If the health education specialist promotes alliances among a number of community agencies with similar interests, this is an example of:

a. collaboration.
b. advocacy.
c. coalition building.
d. community organizing.

146. The purpose of social marketing is to:

a. act on people's behalf.
b. place health issues on the agenda of decision makers.
c. compel others to follow rules, regulations, or ordinances.
d. influence attitudes, beliefs, and practices of a priority population.

147. Which of the following is an example of a cognitive intervention utilized in health teaching?

a. teaching individuals about nutritional food choices.
b. helping individuals understand their fears of living with chronic disease.
c. teaching individuals to carry out specific tasks.
d. reassuring family members that they can care for a disabled child.

148. The section of the research report that is likely to be most significant for readers is the:

a. introduction.
b. results.
c. methods.
d. summary/conclusion.

149. Which of the following is an appropriate intervention for communication with visually impaired individuals?

a. Speak slowly and deliberately.
b. Provide assistive devices, such as letter boards.
c. Speak to the person while approaching.
d. Praise all efforts to communicate.

150. If the health education specialist is interested in applying for a grant to expand health services in a rural health program, which agency may provide a grant?

a. CDC
b. SAMSHA
c. AHRQ
d. HRSA

151. When using Learning-Focused Advocacy Evaluation, the first step is to:

a. outline the purpose of the evaluation.
b. determine the roles and responsibilities.
c. determine a theory of change.
d. determine internal and external measures.

152. The health education specialist has implemented a program to decrease the rate of new HIV/AIDS infections among a largely gay population. All of the following are community-level indicators except:

a. area physicians report a 50% increase in prescriptions for Truvada for pre-exposure prophylaxis (PrEP).
b. free clinics report 10% increase in requests for HIV/AIDS testing.
c. individuals at a clinic report that they believe HIV/AIDS rates have fallen.
d. the public health department reports a 40% decrease in HIV/AIDS infections.

153. Which of the following URL domain extensions should the health education specialist advise individuals is the least valid when searching for information about health?

a. .org
b. .gov
c. .com
d. .mil

154. If the health education specialist is assessing a priority population's need for health-related information and is reviewing economic indicators, such as unemployment rates, the best resource is the:

a. NCHS.
b. DHHS.
c. AHRQ.
d. US Census Bureau.

155. When advocating for change in the delivery of care to older adults, the health education specialist finds that one insurance representative routinely questions the right of the health education specialist to address the issue and claims that no real problems exist. The tactic that the insurance representative is using is:

a. discounting.
b. discrediting
c. dulcifying.
d. deflecting.

156. If an individual is able to slowly read directions out loud but, when questioned, the person clearly does not understand the meaning enough to carry out the directions, the individual would be classified as having:

a. literacy.
b. illiteracy.
c. low literacy.
d. functional illiteracy.

157. Which of the following would be classified as an organizational channel of communication?

a. videos for discussion
b. company newsletter
c. list of questions for individuals to ask physicians
d. speech at a town hall meeting

158. A local television station has agreed to run public service ads for an educational program the health education specialist is implementing in the community. While this would save money for the program, the first question the health education specialist should ask is:

a. "What do you expect in return for running the ads?"
b. "Why do you want to run the ads?"
c. "What hours and how frequently will the ads run?"
d. "Would you also consider becoming a sponsor for the program?"

159. An individual who is paid to actively seek to influence a senator's vote on a public health issue by providing information and statistics is a(n):

a. agitator.
b. advocate.
c. health education specialist.
d. lobbyist.

160. Which of the following websites does NOT provide information about advocacy evaluation?

a. Innovation Network (innonet.org)
b. WK Kellogg Foundation (wkkf.org)
c. The California Endowment (calendow.org)
d. The Evaluation Exchange (hfrp.org)

161. What level of system change is involved when the health education specialist attempts to change the basic mindset or beliefs of individuals regarding how a system works?

a. paradigm
b. system elements
c. system structure
d. goals

162. A free health clinic for Mexican migrant farm workers is located near migrant housing and open from Monday to Friday from 8 AM to 5 PM, but attendance has been very poor. The most likely reason for the poor use of the facility is:

a. fear of Western medicine.
b. hours of business.
c. good health of migrant workers.
d. distrust of free services.

163. When determining the feasibility of implementing recommendations for changes based on a health impact assessment (HIA), which of the following must be considered?

a. multiple factors
b. resources
c. timeline
d. costs

164. Pilot studies should be conducted:

a. in a setting similar to those where the intervention will be used.
b. in mock settings similar to those where the intervention will be used.
c. in order to guarantee the ultimate success of the intervention.
d. in order to test the hypotheses on which the intervention is based.

165. According to the systems approach to organizational change (Rowitz), the first stage is:

a. construct or revise mission and vision statements.
b. clarify values.
c. identify goals and objectives.
d. develop an action plan.

Answer Key and Explanations for Test #2

1. B: An inherent weakness in a system design resulting from inadequate risk management and testing is categorized as a vulnerability. An attack occurs when someone tries to gain access in order to steal information. Risks also include malicious software, which can include viruses, worms, scareware, malware, Trojan horses, spyware, and root kits. People may use phishing to attempt to get individuals to divulge private information or spam, which is bulk messages flooding a site and sometimes introducing malware or viruses.

2. D: Kirkpatrick's four-level training evaluation method comprises the levels of:

- Reaction: This assesses the participant's favorable opinion regarding training.
- Learning: This evaluates the degree to which participants achieved the goals of learning (knowledge, skills, mindset) set out by the program.
- Behavior: This assesses the participants' ability to apply skills/knowledge learned in training to the real world outside of the training.
- Results: This assesses whether targeted outcomes are achieved because of the training and follow-up.

3. A: When assessing the need for health-related information, the initial step is to identify the specific needs so that the information gathered and disseminated is appropriate. Once needs are identified, the need must be matched to the source material and leads pursued to find the necessary information. After information is located, it should be assessed to determine the quality of the information and organized in a manner that it is accessible for the priority population.

4. B: According to the American School Health Association, advanced placement classes are not an aspect of school health (although they may represent quality education). Aspects of school health include nutritious foods, programs of physical activity, adequate and appropriate health education, programs to promote staff health, and student services, such as counseling or psychological and social services. The best practices in school health include active administrative leadership, coordinated and collaborative approach, safe and nurturing learning environment, and adequate commitment of time, staff, and resources.

5. B: If the health specialist chooses a software option for instructional purposes that is the easiest for participants to use but the most difficult for educators because of a complex interface for entering content, the health educations specialist is applying the ethical principle of beneficence because the health education specialist has given priority to the participants' needs. Beneficence is applied when someone acts for the benefit of another. Beneficence should apply to all aspects of a program.

6. D: According to the principle standard of the *National Standards for Culturally and Linguistically Appropriate Services in Health and Health Care*, health care providers should be responsive to "diverse health beliefs and practices, preferred language, health literacy, and other communication needs." Standards 5 through 8 address communication and language assistance and include the need to offer language assistance by trained professional to those with limited English proficiency at no cost and to inform individuals of the availability of language assistance. Multimedia materials and signage should be in the languages in common use within the community.

7. C: If collaboration among a priority population, partners, and other stakeholders is important for the success of an education program, the health education specialist should elicit input during the planning phase from these three groups so that they can begin working together early in the process. When people are part of planning, they are more likely to be engaged, and cooperative efforts that occur during plan development can foster further collaboration once the program is implemented.

8. A: When considering the impact of delivered messages to a priority population, *reach* refers to the number of individuals who see/hear the message and *recall* to the number who remember seeing or hearing the message. If the reach is extensive but the recall is poor (or *vice versa*), then the communication strategy should be reviewed. The impact can also be evaluated according to outcomes (such as increased immunizations after a campaign to increase immunizations) and the number of retweets or "likes" on social media.

9. D: An example of a primary prevention study is assessing decreased rates of influenza after a campaign to increase immunizations. A primary prevention study includes a cause (primary prevention campaign to increase immunizations) and an effect that does not occur (influenza). The change in the community (the indicator) can be inferred indirectly by a decrease in cases of influenza. In some cases, multiple indicators must be selected to determine the effectiveness of primary prevention.

10. A: The primary focus of the Elaboration Likelihood Model of communication is persuasion. Persuasion can be carried out through reasoning or through other means. If a person uses reasoning to come to a conclusion, this is referred to as the process of persuasion through the central route (essentially the use of brain power), but if decisions are made on the basis of less considered thought, such as if influenced by advertising, then this is persuasion through the peripheral route.

11. B: When using an interpreter to communicate with a non-English speaker, the health education specialist should use an interpreter of the same gender if possible, speak in a normal tone of voice, and use a qualified professional interpreter. Statements and questions should not be directed to the interpreter. The health education should speak directly to the non-English speaker even though the interpreter will translate the words. It is important to pause long enough for the interpreter to finish translating because two people speaking may confuse the listener.

12. C: According to the *Federal Plain Language Guidelines*, the sentence that would be preferred is: "The information is for your use." The guidelines suggest that documents should be directed to the individual reader in the second person (you) even though they will be disseminated to a wide audience. Passive voice should be avoided in favor of active, and language should be simple with technical terms defined. If a document is intended for a number of different audiences, then separate documents should be developed.

13. D: The MATCH (Mobilizing Action Toward Community Health) model has five phases that focus on monitoring and evaluating community health and identifying opportunities to improve community health by promoting evidence-based programs and influencing community organizations and community members. Information should be disseminated throughout the community through a variety of means, including media (newspapers, videos, radio), classes, fliers, posters, and other printed material. The five phases include: (1) selecting goals, (2) planning interventions, (3) developing program, (4), preparing or implementation, and (5) evaluating.

14. A: If a needs assessment shows that one community offers more in services to older adults than those offered in another community, the type of needs this represents is relative because it is based on a disparity or lack of equity. However, the actual need may depend on a variety of factors, including demographic differences. Perceived needs are based on what people believe about need. Normative needs are based on custom or consensus. Expressed needs are those that people have voiced.

15. D: According to the CDC's workplace health promotion, when implementing an organizational program to increase breast cancer screening, the best approach to increase mammography screening is one-on-one education. Surveys can help to identify those who have not been adequately screened, but this strategy should be followed by individual contact, such as through face-to-face meetings or telephone contact. Printed or video material may be used as a supplement to one-on-one education and as a subsequent reminder.

16. C: If during data collection, serendipitous findings (accidental discovery of valuable or interesting information) emerge, the best approach is to record the findings for future research. Because modifying a project to take the serendipitous findings into consideration can take appreciable time and study and may significantly alter the project, it is usually best to stay focused on the original project while still collecting all the data for further study. The serendipitous findings should be included in the research report even if the importance of the findings is not clear.

17. B: The maximum number of words per slide when using projection software, such as PowerPoint, should be 50 words, using the largest possible font to make reading easier for those at a distance from the slide. The slide text should be used to highlight important points rather than to outline an entire lecture. The colors used for text should have a high level of contrast to the background, and bright background colors should be avoided.

18. A: If a health education specialist who is working with a predominately Muslim population must set up a series of appointments with individuals and specifically schedules appointments between prayer times so that the appointments do not interfere with their religious practice, this is an example of cultural care preservation. Cultural care preservation refers to providing assistance and care to individuals while still enabling them to maintain their cultural/religious practices without interference.

19. C: A professional development plan could include reading professional journal articles, authoring a journal article, and making a conference presentation about health education. Although reading about health education needs in the popular press may provide valuable insight and may serve as the basis for intervention, this type of reading is not considered part of professional development because the information has not been peer-reviewed and may, at times, be inaccurate or mischaracterized.

20. B: The Boolean operator that should be used most sparingly is NOT. Because this operator eliminates documents that contain a specific term, NOT may eliminate too many documents because the eliminated word may be used as a passing reference in a document with a different focus. There are only three Boolean operators: OR, AND, and NOT. The Boolean operator OR is used to locate similar or synonymous concepts while AND is used to find documents that contain more than one specified term.

21. D: Map charts, such as Graph 1, are an excellent means of displaying data that cover a broad area, such as a number of counties or states. In this case, the numerical data is printed on each component (state) in the map, but the data are categorized (≤400, 400.1—600, and >600) to make interpretation easier. The different categories on a map chart should be color-coded or shaded so that they can be identified easily—usually the higher the category, the brighter or darker the color/shading. It is easy to see on this chart that the Southeast has the highest rates of gonorrhea.

22. B: If utilizing data in Graph 1 (map of the United States showing rates of gonorrhea among women aged 15-24), the data would be considered secondary, which is classified according to the entity that collected the data. If researchers collect their own data directly, such as through surveys and interviews, this is primary data. However, if the researchers utilize data that has been collected by another researcher or entity, then this data is secondary.

23. A: According to Graph 1, the health education specialist can conclude that the Northwest has the lowest rates of gonorrhea. Because the statistics are based on the number of cases per 100,000, low population does not affect the rate. The state with the lowest rate of gonorrhea is New Hampshire (34) in the Northeast, which includes states with low rates and high rates. One cannot assume that the Northwest has better sex education than other states without further research because other factors may be at play.

24. D: When conducting qualitative research, the literature review may be deferred until after all data are collected to avoid the review influencing the research. If data are collected first, then these data can be compared with the data from the literature review to determine where the data differ. The timing of the review of literature may vary depending on the type of qualitative research, and authorities differ on the optimal timing. For example, with ethnographic and historical research, the literature review is usually conducted at the beginning of the research process.

25. A: The HIPAA privacy rule protects individually identifiable health information by outlining the conditions under which it can be utilized for research. Health information that has been deidentified can be utilized without further restrictions. However, in order to use individually identifiable health information, the person must give informed consent unless a waiver has been granted by an IRB or privacy board to utilize information without consent; however, a number of conditions must be met in order to obtain a waiver.

26. B: A culture audit most often begins with surveys. The purpose of a culture audit is to assess the perceptions and values of an organization. A culture audit often explores workers' job satisfaction with questions about whether they believe they are treated fairly and compensated adequately. The first stage of a culture audit is assessment, and this should be followed by analysis of the results and recommendations for changes.

27. C: Obtaining and documenting consent is an indication of ethical rigor when determining the validity of qualitative research. Participants should be aware of the research being conducted and should be informed of their rights and assured that these rights will be protected by the researchers. Ethical rigor is threatened when consent is not obtained, when participants are unaware of their rights or their rights are not protected, or the research reveals the identity of participants.

28. A: When determining the time frame and steps needed to collect data, the best solution may be to conduct a pilot study to assess how long it takes to collect data from subjects and to carry out the necessary data collection procedures. A pilot study can help identify problems that might arise. Data collection often takes two to three times longer than estimated times, and researchers commonly underestimate the time needed.

29. B: The first task in data collection is selecting subjects. Subjects may be selected randomly or specifically chosen based on some criteria. Once the subjects are selected, the other tasks related to data collection occur simultaneously rather than sequentially. Research controls must ensure that data are collected systematically and that there is consistency and accuracy in collection. Problems may occur at any point during data collection and must be attended to promptly.

30. D: An example of a potential research subject that would most likely be classified as having diminished autonomy is an individual diagnosed with bipolar disorder. People with diminished autonomy are classified as vulnerable and in need of extra protection in research. This group of individuals includes those with mental illness or severe physical illness. Others classified as having diminished autonomy include neonates, human fetuses, people with severe developmental disorders, children, and prisoners. While these individuals may be older than 65 years of age, non-English speaking, or have a condition such as an amputation, these characteristics alone do not deem one to have diminished autonomy. Those with diminished autonomy should still be able to make a choice to the extent of their ability.

31. A: The best method to follow in order to plan for technical failure is to routinely back up files. Backup may be done to a secure server, to cloud storage, to an external hard drive, or to a portable memory device, such as a flash drive. Backups should ideally be done each day and set to record automatically. Despite adequate maintenance and troubleshooting, equipment failure can still occur. Storing only to a portable memory device poses a problem if the device is lost or damaged.

32. C: The first step in obtaining an appropriate data collection instrument for a large-scale study is to conduct a literature review, paying particular attention to the instruments used to collect data. While an instrument can be designed specifically for a research project, with a large-scale project, questions of validity and reliability may arise if the instrument has not been properly evaluated and validated. Additionally, designing an appropriate tool may be a lengthy process.

33. A: When collecting data about rates of influenza, a good source of secondary data is the CDC, which collects data about communicable diseases. Secondary data are those that are collected by others. Secondary data are available through many government agencies, insurance companies, universities, foundations, and professional associations. Census data is also secondary data and provides demographic information. One advantage of secondary data is that much data is available free of cost and is easily obtainable.

34. B: Needs assessments are completed to determine the needs for an educational program. If, for example, a needs assessment determines whether children in the community are immunized against whooping cough, the type of need this focuses on is normative. Normative needs are based on standards or levels that are determined by experts or authorities, such as the governmental agencies. Normative needs exist if a group or community does not meet the established standards.

35. D: If the health education specialist wants to measure the self-confidence of adolescents participating in a risk-reduction program, in order to have content validity (logical validity), the health education specialist must first define the domain. That is, the health education specialist must determine all the criteria that represent self-confidence because the testing must measure the correct content if the results are to have significance. Because there is a subjective element to selecting criteria, testing bias may occur.

36. C: The PRECEDE-PROCEED model, which is used for healthcare planning, has three phases for PRECEDE and five for PROCEED. During the PRECEED portion, which is preparation for implementation, three different assessments are carried out: social, epidemiological, and educational/ecological. During the PROCEED portion, administrative and policy assessment is done to identify resources followed by implementation. The last three phases are evaluations, including process evaluation, impact evaluation, and (last) outcomes evaluation.

37. B: Smoking cessation is likely to have the most impact on health because smoking is associated with so many adverse effects, including hypertension, heart disease, COPD, and lung cancer. When conducting needs assessments, one of the methods of prioritizing the identified needs is to consider the impact of intervention as well as compliance. While smoking cessation has a large positive effect on health, adherence is often poor, and this must be a consideration as well.

38. A: While CHES certification is voluntary, the purpose of receiving the CHES certification is to demonstrate mastery of necessary skills across all practice areas. These practice areas include the following settings: community, school, health care, business/industry college/university, and college/university health services. CHES certification requires health education academic preparation, passing a written exam, and completion of 75 hours of continuing education contact hours over a 5-year period.

39. C: When conducting a needs assessment utilizing the three-phase model (explore, gather/analyze data, and make decisions), the first phase (explore) includes identifying areas of concern as well as preparing a management plan, considering potential sources for data, and deciding on measurable indicators. The second phase (gather/analyze data) includes not only gathering and analyzing data but also determining the target population, prioritizing needs, and summarizing the results of data analysis. The third phase (make decisions) includes identifying possible solutions, prioritizing and selecting solutions, and developing an action plan and preparing a report.

40. D: When utilizing a strategy grid to prioritize, and *need* and *cost* are the criteria selected, the category that has the highest priority is probably high need/low cost because cost is usually a concern. However, in some cases, an intervention that is categorized as high need/high cost may be the first choice if economically feasible. The strategy grid typically is a square divided into 4 sections, and the interventions are placed in the squares depending on how they fit the selected criteria.

41. A: If a community is faced with high rates of adolescent pregnancy, and the health education specialist is planning a high school educational program to prevent pregnancy in collaboration with the school district, the most critical element to consider is policy. Because the participants will be minors and because there are religious and cultural implications to preventing pregnancy, the health education specialist should review state as well as school district policies regarding sex education, which can vary widely. Some districts, for example, may allow only abstinence education while others provide condoms.

42. C: If a number of key individuals in the community have been vociferous in their disapproval of the program, believing it will result in increased promiscuity, and have influenced others to oppose the program, the communication theory that this exemplifies is the contagion theory. This theory postulates that when a majority (or a smaller group of influential people) has a position about an issue, many others will simply take the same position without real consideration of the issues involved.

43. B: The primary goal of the Directors of Health Promotion and Education (DHPE) is health equity through influencing health policy and systems change and increasing the capacity of public health. DHPE allows members to exchange information and best practices, advocates for policy changes to promote health equity, collaborates with other agencies, provides support for community analysis, and provides health equity tools. DHPE offers internship and fellowships for students of minority-serving institutions to gain experience working in public health programs.

44. D: Socioeconomic status has the most influence on health behaviors while religion, place of residence, and race have less influence. Socioeconomic status may have a positive or negative effect on health behavior with positive effects correlating directly to higher socioeconomic status and negative effects to lower. Other factors that influence health behavior are age, gender, and the type of social support system that is available. Advanced age and poor social support systems are associated with negative health behaviors.

45. B: If the trend toward increased use of e-cigarettes continues, the impact on health is likely to be negative. While many people believe that e-cigarettes are less harmful and may help smokers quit smoking, in fact the high levels of nicotine pose health risks, and studies show that e-cigarettes do not help people quit smoking because the smokers remain addicted to nicotine. Of particular concern is the marked increase in use of e-cigarettes among adolescents.

46. A: When attempting to engage a priority population in participating in assessment, the best method is likely to show how participants benefit by participating. Paying people will attract a certain subgroup of people, but these may not be representative. Appealing to social consciousness may be a motivation for some people as well, but again the group may not be representative. Applying punitive measures for non-participation is a type of coercion and is not ethical.

47. C: A mission statement generally reflects the current status and is essentially an organization's statement of purpose. The mission statement is developed on the basis of data and analysis of the program. The mission statement, which is usually one sentence or a short paragraph, should describe the organization's role within the community. The mission statement is often followed by a more complete explanation, which may include statements of philosophy and values and may also describe the history of the organization.

48. C: When preparing a visual display showing the results of a needs assessment for a presentation to community representatives, the best method of display is a pie chart. The pie chart is the simplest display because there is no X and Y axis to interpret. The pie chart may be color-coded for ease of interpretation, and the pie chart itself may be labeled rather than using a legend. The pie chart works best if there are only a few categories.

49. A: The database that is likely to provide the best information about school health and school-aged children is Education Resources Information Center (ERIC). ERIC is a good source for journals as well as reports of proceedings from conferences, which may not be available from other sources. ERIC is sponsored by the US Department of Education, Institute of Education Sciences. Searches can be limited to peer-reviewed journals only and to articles with full-text availability. Searches can use quotation marks and field: term syntax.

50. C: The three domains of learning, which are used to categorize, plan, and evaluate learning, are:

- Cognitive: knowledge, comprehension, application, analysis, synthesis, and evaluation (thinking domain)
- Affective: receiving, responding, valuing, organizing, and characterizing (feeling domain)
- Psychomotor: perception, responding, acting, adaptation, and origination (skills domain)

The three domains are interdependent and can be activated simultaneously as part of the learning experience. Effective teaching should be focused on all three domains.

51. A: When considering the frame of mind of participants in an educational program in relation to readiness to learn, frame of mind usually involves concern with the present. Therefore, it is important to focus on how the educational program can affect the participant's current situation rather than focusing solely on future outcomes, especially when working with populations from the lower socioeconomic levels because these populations often have to, by necessity, focus on daily concerns, such as adequate food and housing.

52. C: If the goal of data collection is to assess participant satisfaction with education provided in a community-wide program, the best initial method is probably surveying. Surveys can be completed by participants during the program or at the end, and are relatively inexpensive and easy to administer. Especially when a large population is involved, interviews may be time consuming, and it can be difficult to achieve a representative sample. Records review is not likely to reflect satisfaction, although attendance may give some indication. Focus groups may be better for planning than for assessing satisfaction.

53. D: An example of a well-written objective is this statement: "Following a class on smoking cessation, the participants will be able to list 4 health risks associated with smoking." This statement includes (1) the condition/testing situation (following a class in smoking cessation), (2) the learner (the participants), (3) expected behavior or performance (will be able to), and (4) the criterion to exhibit mastery (list 4 health risks associated with smoking).

54. B: Based on Graph 2, the greatest change in average weekly hours playing video games occurred between ages 10 and 11, the period in which the child moves from childhood into preadolescence. Children at this age often gain more independence and have less direct supervision, so the parents may not be aware of the actual number of hours that children spend playing video games, especially since many children now have video games in their rooms and can play undetected by their parents or caregivers.

55. D: Considering the results of the survey illustrated in Graph 2, if planning an educational program to highlight the importance of decreasing hours of video game playing, an educational program should target the parents to increase awareness of their children's video gaming habits and to stress the importance of ensuring that children have limited access to video games and more opportunities for physical activities. Parents should be advised about parental controls for TV, video gaming consoles, and computers.

56. D: Physical readiness to learn is most affected by task complexity. The more complex the task, the more difficult it may be to physically carry out the steps required. Tasks that require fine motor skills are generally more difficult than those that require gross motor skills. Other factors that may affect physical readiness include the person's health status, gender (including such issues as body size, musculature, and center of gravity), measures of ability, and environmental effects (such as extreme cold or heat).

57. C: According to Healthy People 2030, transportation options are considered social determinants of health, which are situations within the person's environment that may directly or indirectly influence health. Other social determinants of health include access to health care, education, and employment opportunities, and the availability of services and social support within the community. Some social factors, such as high rates of crime or violence, may especially have negative effects on people's health.

58. D: The focus of a goal statement should be on end results or the ideal that an organization wants to reach at the end of a process rather than current practice or process. A goal should be feasible, or it is not realistic. A goal is usually stated in fairly broad or general terms, such as "lowering costs of health care" or "improving patient satisfaction." Goals are supported by a number of objectives, which generally describe the specific actions to be carried out in order to reach the goal.

59. B: When preparing written materials regarding health matters for a community group, the materials should generally be written at about the fifth-grade level, assuming that the priority population will include those with a range in literacy. The text should generally avoid long, complex sentences and medical jargon, although applying strict readability formulas (which usually advise short sentences) may be counterproductive. The most important factor is that the writing be clear, easy to understand, and contain vocabulary with which the reader is familiar.

60. A: If designing an educational program about mental health issues for Middle Eastern immigrants, the best course title is probably "Steps to Better Health" because there is considerable social stigma attached to mental illness in most Middle Eastern cultures, so people may not be willing to attend a program with a more direct course title. People who are depressed or have other signs of emotional or mental distress often have somatic complaints, such as headaches or stomachaches, and often resist counseling or therapy, preferring medications instead.

61. C: A geographic factor to consider when identifying a priority population is the community, city, area of the country, or state in which the population resides. A population may also be identified by location at which the population can be reached, such as a specific school, church, or organization. Demographic information, such as age, gender, level of income, level of education, and marital status, may also be used to identify a priority population.

62. D: The ethical principle that is applied when members of the priority population are encouraged to help determine the type of educational program that they need is autonomy, which refers to the right to self-determination. Veracity refers to honesty and truth telling. Beneficence is the ethical principle that requires that actions be taken for the purpose of doing good. Nonmaleficence refers to the ethical principle that actions should do no harm (although sometimes an action may cause harm as a means to achieve good, such as with chemotherapy).

63. C: If the health education specialist focuses on building relationships within the community and establishing collaboration and power sharing among agencies, this type of leadership is transactional. Transformational leadership focuses on changing the system and coming up with new ideas while organizational leadership focuses on managing and solving problems and encouraging others. Strategic leadership focuses on achieving goals through strategic planning with an orientation toward the future.

64. B: If an educational program about diabetic prevention targeting Mexican immigrant farmworker families has been meeting at the public health offices, but participation has been very low, the best place to consider moving the classes is to churches in the community. Mexican Americans as a group tend to be religious (often Catholic) and feel comfortable in the church environment. They may feel intimidated by other environments, such as employment offices or community colleges, especially if they are undocumented or speak little English.

65. C: If the health education specialist has planned a group activity for a class period but participants refuse to cooperate, the best response is to try a different approach. The planned group activity may have cultural implications that the education specialist does not understand, and forcing people to participate in an activity that they have rejected serves little purpose. A health education specialist should always be flexible and prepared to modify lesson plans to meet the needs of the participants.

66. A: The sound that is likely to have the most negative effect on learning is intermittent noise from nearby construction. People tend to accommodate to steady noise—such as the hum of the air conditioning unit, background music, or traffic sounds—and no longer notice it after a time unless it is overwhelmingly noisy. However, intermittent sounds are less predictable, and they are much more difficult to block from consciousness and may be very disruptive to a class.

67. D: In order to be ADA compliant when planning a program, plans must be made to accommodate service animals, personal aides, and wheelchairs. The only service animals recognized by the ADA are dogs and in special cases miniature horses. Accommodations are not required for other animals. Additionally, comfort animals are not included as part of ADA regulations, but some states may have provisions regarding comfort animals. People often believe that comfort animals are classified the same as service animals, which have been trained to carry out specific tasks.

68. B: When preparing a media bite as part of a campaign of media advocacy to promote an educational program, the media bite should be 7-15 seconds long. The media bite should be a brief description that outlines the main purpose that should be conveyed to the public. The media bite should be written to appeal to the public and to catch attention, so it may include humor or an appeal to reason or emotion.

69. A: With the CDCynergy model of program planning, before developing communication strategies, it is necessary to identify/profile the priority population. The model has 6 different phases, beginning with definition and description of the problem followed by analysis and identifying/profiling the priority population. At this point, communication strategies should be developed and then a plan for evaluation and implementation as well as methods for receiving feedback.

70. C: Qualitative methods of assessment are usually part of formative evaluation and done to help to understand needs, to clarify the theories on which the project is based, and to improve the project. Formative evaluation is done before project development through literature review and analysis of problems and stakeholders. During the development of the project, evaluation may help to drive the development, identifying areas of problem. Formative evaluation may continue during implementation with focus groups and interviews, and may be done as part of ongoing monitoring.

71. B: When eliciting input about a health education plan targeting homeless veterans in an inner city, the organization that may be most helpful is likely the Department of Veterans Affairs, which has numerous programs already in place to assist homeless veterans. Programs include housing and employment assistance. Wounded Warriors focuses on military members who have been injured and their families. The Salvation Army has many programs for the homeless in general. The VFW is a fraternal organization with charitable and educational programs.

72. D: The most important factor in facilitating collaboration efforts among priority population, partners, and other stakeholders is demonstrating areas of shared concern because this focuses on the present rather than potential future benefits, which may be harder to appreciate. It is generally preferable to focus on the positives of collaboration than the negatives of lack of collaboration because coerced collaboration is rarely successful.

73. B: While all of these methods may prove helpful, in order to obtain data about the impact of heroin use on the local community, the health education specialist will most likely need to conduct primary data collection unless another local agency has already carried this out. Secondary data may provide state and national statistics that can be useful for benchmarks but are usually not adequate for local areas. Observations may be part of primary data collection.

74. C: If a group of community members opposes programs to help homeless veterans because the members believe that the veterans are looking for a handout because they do not want to work, as an advocate, the best response is to reframe the issue. If reframing, the health education specialist should not attempt to repudiate the claims or ask for evidence but should discuss alternative issues, such as the lack of adequate support programs and lack of employment opportunities.

75. D: When creating SMART objectives/goals, SMART stands for:

- Specific: Explain what, where, and why the objectives/goals are needed.
- Measurable: Include measures that will determine when objectives/goals are met.
- Attainable: Develop realistic objective/goals that are sustainable.
- Relevant: Connect objectives/goals to mission and vision statements.
- Timely/Time-bound: Establish objectives goals when needed and target dates for reaching objectives/goals.

76. A: The learning method that is likely to result in the greatest retention is practicing/restating. Learners should, for example, be encouraged to do return demonstrations when learning to carry out an action. A good way to help learners retain information is to have them teach the information to others, such as through class presentations or creation of audiovisual materials. Repetition is especially important for retention, especially if information is to move from short-term memory to long-term.

77. B: When using a logic model to plan an education program, participants' ability to list adverse effects of nicotine would be considered a short-term outcome because it relates to knowledge and/or skills acquired during the intervention. Changes in behavior, on the other hand, such as decreased rate of smoking after 6 months, is an intermediate outcome. Long-term outcomes are those that relate to morbidity and mortality, such as decreased incidence of bronchitis and cough and decreased rate of COPD/lung cancer after 20 years.

78. C: The best way to integrate health teaching into a drop-in clinic where large numbers of patients often experience extended waiting periods is by providing video presentations. The presentations should be relatively short (5-10 minutes) so that patients and family members can often view the entire presentation, and the presentations should be closed captioned in case the waiting area is noisy and the video is difficult to hear. The video presentation may be supplemented by posters and pamphlets. Audio recordings are the least likely to be successful because of noise interference.

79. A: Media attention (newspapers, TV, radio, magazines) is not likely to hinder implementation of an educational program and may, in fact, foster support through educating the priority population. Factors that may hinder implementation include lack of community support, inadequate funding, inadequate resources, limited planning time, and lack of coordination. Another important factor that hinders implementation is a health education specialist who is charged with implementing a program but has too many other projects to handle, leaving too little time.

80. D: If the health education specialist has developed an educational program that will be implemented by members and volunteers at a service agent, everyone involved in implementation has the responsibility to ensure that ethical principles are applied to the implementation process, not just the professional staff who are expected to comply with professional codes of ethics. During the training process for staff and volunteers, the importance of applying ethical principles should be addressed directly so that everyone is clear about expectations.

81. B: If an education program is to be implemented as part of a research study, the participants should sign informed consent documents prior to participation and should have a clear understanding of the type of research to be carried out and how any information about the individuals will be utilized. Participants should also be advised that they have the right to discontinue participation at any time and assured that their confidentiality will be respected.

82. C: If, prior to the first phase of implementation of a new program, a review of the budget shows that the funds for implementation are insufficient, and no further sources of funds can be identified, the best solution is to scale back the program. This may mean to eliminate parts of the program, use less expensive materials and equipment, change venues, or use a phase-in approach. Planning should be based on secured funds rather than potential funds, and the budgetary requirements should be considered during all stages of planning.

83. A: When recruiting individuals needed for implementation of an education plan, the primary concern is that the individuals' skills match those needed. The job description should be very detailed, and the individuals' applications reviewed in relation to that description. While good communications skills are important, they will not help if the individuals lack skills to do the job. The individuals' relationship to the priority population may or may not be significant, and care must be used in assessing physical and emotional health to comply with ADA regulations.

84. C: Creation of a nonprofit organization is a self-sustaining source of funding for securing resources needed to implement an education plan. Nonprofit organizations have ongoing requests for donations or activities to increase income, which can then be distributed to the program rather than returned to investors. Grants, whether public (such as state or federal) or private (such as from companies), are usually time-limited and may be provided on a one-time basis or may be reapplied for periodically, such as every year.

85. C: If researching the efficacy of the different types of teaching approaches for a health education program, the database that may provide access to the most applicable information is ERIC (Education Resources Information Center). ERIC is sponsored by the US Department of Education, the Institute of Education Sciences. ERIC provides bibliographic information as well as links to full texts of many articles. Searches can use direct quotations, field:term syntax, and Boolean operators.

86. D: This question would be classified as mutually exclusive because each answer is distinct and does not overlap with other answers. However, the questions would be classified as not collectively exhaustive because the choices do not include all means of hearing about the program, such as by word of mouth or by the radio. In order to ensure that selections are collectively exhaustive, researchers often include a choice of "other" and allow the participants to write in other choices.

87. A: Based on the CDC chart (Graph 3), showing the percentage of adults in the United States receiving influenza vaccinations between 1997 and March 2015, the age group that has shown the least improvement in rates since 1997 is the 65 and older group. While this group has the highest overall rate of vaccinations, the rate in 1997 was approximately 65% and 70% in 2015, a 5% increase. By contrast, the 50-64 age group increased approximately 20% and the 18-49 age group by approximately 15%.

88. C: If using the data in graph 3 to determine the priority population to target for education about influenza vaccinations, the education is likely to provide best long-term outcomes if targeted to the 18-49 age group. This group has the lowest percentage of vaccinations across the board. Additionally, since this is the youngest age group, changing vaccination habits in this group should carry over into the older age group as time passes and the participants move into the 50-64 age group.

89. A: If creating a GANTT chart as a tool for time and project management, the first step is to create a project plan identifying tasks and order of completion so that the activities can be placed sequentially in the Y-axis of the chart and the times on the X-axis. Some times and activities may overlap, and this will be clearly evident. The GANTT chart can be easily modified if created with a computer program as estimated times and even activities may need to be revised during the course of the project.

90. C: If a pilot study showed that even though the participants resisted the method of instruction and complained, the health education specialist persisted in using the same method, assuming the participants would later see the value of the method, this could be considered a barrier to learning. The health education specialist must consider the priority population—age, gender, and culture—when planning methods of instruction and should be prepared to modify delivery if the participants do not respond adequately.

91. B: If, as part of a marketing plan for a health education program, informational literature is sent out to community members who have previously attended health education classes, this is an example of a targeted message aimed at a subgroup of people (those who previously attended classes). Targeted messages are aimed at groups while tailored messages are aimed at individuals, so targeted messages may be less effective than tailored because of the heterogeneous nature of groups, even those with similar interests or experiences.

92. D: If a state has limited Medicaid expansion, leaving many low-income citizens without insurance or access to medical care, this is an example of a health determinant. Health determinants are those factors, such as access to medical care, that influence health. Health determinants may include a wide range of factors. Policies may limit or allow access, social factors may encourage or discourage health practices, health services may or may not be available, individual behavior may promote or interfere with health, and biology/genetics may lead to resistance to disease or development of disease.

93. A: If assessing reactions of the participants to a training session in order to modify the course as needed, quantifiable results may best be obtained with a Likert scale, which is a bipolar scaling method in which participants select a number on a scale showing how much they agree or disagree with a statement. If the scale contains an even number, then there is no midpoint and each answer must skew either positive or negative. The Likert scale gives a greater range than yes/no questions and is more easily quantifiable than interviews and open-ended questions.

94. C: If a focus group of inner-city adolescents in a drug treatment program answered questions about drug use, and based on the results of this focus group, a health education plan is to be developed for the county, including a large rural area, the greatest concern is generalizability. To be generalizable, findings must extend from the focus group to the larger population, but the social and economic status of the adolescents in the inner city may be quite different from those in the rural area, and access to drugs may be different as well.

95. B: If a health education specialist is developing a web-based interactive educational program for a federal agency, Section 508 (technical standards) of the Rehabilitation Act requires that the website have text/audio descriptions of any visual display, including pictures, illustrations, and videos. Software must be accessible, and accessibility applications, such as screen readers and Braille displays, must be supported. While Section 508 does not apply to non-federal organizations and is not required of those receiving grants, it is a good marketing and ethical strategy to follow the federal regulations.

96. D: If the health education specialist at a community hospital is utilizing SWOT (strength-weakness-opportunities-threats) analysis to review an educational program about heart health for a primarily low-income population and finds that the community location where the classes are held is no longer on the public transportation bus route, this information would be classified as a threat. While the program itself may be strong, a low-income population may rely on public transportation, so the fact that the location is no longer served by buses may decrease the number of participants.

97. B: If the health education specialist is planning advocacy intervention as part of a public health program to reduce the rates of obesity in children and adolescents, asking the board of education to improve the school lunch program is an example of advocacy intervention at the systems level. Advocacy at the community level includes working with school principals to eliminate soft drinks from vending machines. Advocacy at the individual level includes meeting with families to discuss their children's activities and meeting with children to discuss the need for exercise.

98. A: If the health education specialist has devised a number of interventions to increase use of a well-baby clinic and the interventions are to be carried out by public health staff, in order to ensure intervention fidelity, an essential element in the program is training. In order to evaluate response to the interventions, they must be used consistently and in the same manner. The health education specialist should prepare an implementation guide that outlines the process involved and may also conduct seminars and practice sessions with role playing.

99. B: If an electronic monitoring device transmits data, such as BP and pulse, daily or with a regular frequency, and the data can be accessed in list form and displayed in line graphs over the internet from secure servers, this type of data is referred to as trend data because it shows how the vital signs trend over a period of time. This type of data collection is being used increasingly as monitoring devices become less intrusive and more compact. The data are often transmitted through Bluetooth technology so the person can remain mobile.

100. A: If the electronic monitoring devices are only available to participants who can afford to purchase them and manual recordings must be made by other participants, the ethical principle that has been breached is equity. Equity requires that all participants have equal access and equal opportunities, but those with the electronic monitoring devices clearly have an advantage in terms of recording, reporting, and feedback. A lack of equity in a project can result in difficulty assessing outcomes.

101. D: When designing a program for delivery of educational material, it is important to understand the population. While many of the older generation are computer literate, this population often is less comfortable with computer-assisted or internet instruction than younger generations who grew up with computers. In this case, the best solution is probably to hold orientation classes to walk people through the use of the computer-assisted instructional modules. Additionally, printed instructions should be available for people to refer to later.

102. C: If the health education specialist is advocating for a program to reduce obesity in children and adolescents and believes that billboards for high-sugar soft drinks in the area are targeting minority children, the first step is to survey all billboards to gather evidence. The survey should contain photo evidence and should note the contents of the ads and the locations. When making claims, it is essential that the health education specialist have factual information rather than anecdotal.

103. B: If gap analysis is being used as part of capacity assessment, the focus is on identifying deficiencies that exist between the current performance and a desired performance or future goal. Gap analysis may identify situations in which resources are not used to their full potential. Also, if a program wants to expand, for example, from providing 3 services to 6 services, gap analysis should identify what would be needed to make this transition in terms of resources, time, staff, or other elements.

104. C: If a number of activities have been identified as part of development of a Critical Path Method (CPM) work plan, the next step is to identify predecessors and successors. A predecessor is an activity that must be completed before another activity. A successor is an activity that must be completed after another activity. When building the activity-on-arc (AOA) diagram, which utilizes numbered nodes (activities), those activities for which there are no predecessors come directly off of node one.

105. D: A blood pressure cuff is an example of a high-fidelity simulation. High-fidelity simulations include real materials (such as various types of equipment) or realistic materials (such as mannequins used to practice CPR). Activities that require actions and manipulations, such as taking blood pressure or administering shocks with an AED, are very difficult to learn without the use of real or realistic equipment. Low-fidelity simulation includes printed materials, verbally presented information, and audiotapes.

106. C: If the health education specialist must teach staff members to master a number of tasks related to phasing in of new equipment, the best method to employ is just-in-time presentations as the participants need the information. Especially with equipment that is being phased in, teaching in advance of use is of little value because the participants will likely need to be retrained because of inadequate retention. Just-in-time presentations are often used when participants must master specific tasks.

107. A: If, when collaborating with others in the development of an education plan, the health education specialist presents a potential decision about the project and then makes a final decision based on input from other members of the team, this exemplifies the participatory style of leadership. With the democratic style, the group comes up with a solution but the leader makes the final decision. With consultative, the leader makes a decision, welcomes input, but rarely changes the decision. With the bureaucratic style, the leader rigidly follows rules and decision making and expects everyone else to do so.

108. B: Analyzing large amounts of data in order to identify underlying patterns is referred to as data mining. This process is often done automatically with software applications. Data mining, for example, may identify groups of data with similarities that can lead to further analysis. Data mining may be used with multiple records, such as when searching patients' electronic health records for specific types of responses as part of research. Data mining includes the detection of anomalies, identification of relationships, clustering of data, classification of data, regression, and summarization.

109. B: If a health education specialist is monitoring national rates of rehospitalization of psychiatric patients and comparing them with internal rates of an institution, this is an example of external benchmarking. When using external benchmarking to make decisions about a program, it is important that the definitions used be the same for the national rates and the internal rates, and that the population and risk stratification be the same; otherwise, the data can be misleading.

110. D: If a community agency writes an article for free about an educational program in its print and digital newsletter even though the program is not affiliated with the agency, this is an example of earned media because the promotion is earned by virtue of quality or reputation but does not involve cost. Earned media is essentially free promotion outside of the traditional advertising venues. Earned media may occur through letters to the editor, editorial comments, and published results of surveys or polls citing the program.

111. A: If the health education specialist is developing a memorandum of understanding (MOU) with another agency in order to implement a joint project, the most important thing to remember about an MOU is that it is a legal contract. Because of this, the MOU should be reviewed by an attorney with experience in contracts, and the terms of the agreement—including financial arrangements, parties involved, responsibilities, shared liabilities, and disclaimers—should be clearly outlined.

112. B: When choosing strategies for program implementation, the health education specialist should review the literature to ensure that each strategy has efficacy. That is, the strategy should produce the expected outcomes. Because each program is in some way different from other programs, it is important to assess the strategy as it has been used in similar programs because what works in one situation may not be effective in another. The strategy used should be carefully reassessed during implementation and after to determine if modification is needed.

113. A: An example of a workplace implementation of an intervention at the individual level is providing a financial bonus for not smoking. Individual strategies focus on the individual's lifestyle and can include health behaviors, risk factors, and/or health status. Other types of strategies may focus on interpersonal elements (such as development of a mentoring program), organizational (such as a smoking cessation program), or environmental (such as improved lighting and sound reduction). A combination of strategies is often most effective.

114. C: According to the CDC's Steps to Wellness, the first step to implementing a comprehensive wellness program in a workplace focusing on physical activity is to build support for the plan. Building support requires the identification of champions in the workplace who can lead by example to promote the health benefits of activity. Interested staff members should be identified because these individuals can serve on a wellness committee to identify activities and promote participation. The next steps include to planning and assessing, promoting the plan, and finally implementing the plan.

115. D: A physical activity program is most likely to be an effective adjunct to a program to prevent, identify, and treat depression. Physical activity helps to instill a sense of well-being and has been effective in treating mild depression. Specific lifestyle activities, such as participating in exercises with other members of the organization, may be recommended for the individual. In some cases, depression may be exacerbated by substance abuse, so referrals to substance abuse programs should be made as needed.

116. B: When analyzing data, frequency distribution can be computed with nominal data, but percentile, addition and subtraction, mean and median, standard deviation, and ratio cannot. Nominal data are qualitative in that nominal scales involve naming or labeling, such as choices indicating eye color or gender. Thus, the frequency of a number of choices (16 males and 14 females, for example) can be calculated but the condition of being one choice or another (male or female) cannot be quantified.

117. A: According to Graph 4, the age group in which there is the least difference in heavy drinking between males and females is 18-24. In this age group, females have at least 1 heavy drinking day in the year at a rate that is 80% that of males (a 20% difference). In the other age groups, the difference ranges from about 50% to 65% with males the heaviest drinkers—the highest rate is for males in the 25-44 age group and the lowest in the 65 and older group. Female reports of heavy drinking remain fairly stable from ages 18-24 but decrease markedly in the 45-64 age group and even further in the 65 and older group.

118. A: Assessing outcomes to determine whether they were intended or not is part of impact evaluation, which evaluates whether the program reached its goals as projected. Impact evaluation may be carried out at specific times during operation of a program or at the end of a program or period of implementation. Impact evaluation is often conducted to determine policy decisions or to make decisions regarding further financing of a project. Choosing a method of evaluation is an important first step and may include selection of comparison groups.

119. C: When selecting items from an existing instrument, the most important factor to consider is validity in order to ensure that the items measure the intended domain. The health education specialist must be concerned with both internal (results are true for one population) and external validity (results from one population can extend to another population). Face validity, the degree to which an instrument appears to measure the appropriate domain, is not a measure of true validity and should not substitute for rigorous evaluation.

120. B: If an existing instrument includes the item, "How frequently do you use communication media (telephone, telegram, FAX) to communicate with friends and family?" an appropriate modification would be "How frequently do you use communication media (telephone, Facebook, Twitter, Instagram, instant messaging, Skype/FaceTime) to communicate with friends and family?" because the basic structure and focus of the question remains the same, but the examples of communication methods have been updated to reflect more current technology.

121. A: When data from surveys are to be entered into the computer, the health education specialist must first check the data and resolve problems. For example, the health education specialist must decide how to deal with missing data from a subject or excess data, such as when a subject makes two selections instead of one. If subjects must write in a response, such as an occupation, then the selections should be coded before data entry to ensure accuracy and consistency.

122. D: When considering different methods of collecting survey data, the health education specialist recognizes that the benefits of emailed online surveys includes lower risk of error, cost-effectiveness, and convenience but does not include high rates of response. In fact, the response rate for online surveys is often quite low because subjects may ignore the survey because of the number of unwanted emails that people receive. Participation rates may increase if subjects are made aware of the survey in advance and have agreed to participate.

123. B: The purpose of establishing an institutional review board (IRB) in research involving human subjects is oversight/monitoring to ensure that ethical, scientific, and regulatory standards are met. The IRB is charged with ensuring that the participants' rights are protected, that informed consent was obtained using appropriate methods, and that the benefits of participation outweigh the risks. The IRB determines if research is exempt from review, requires expedited review, or requires complete review.

124. C: The section of a research report that usually contains descriptions that include words, numbers, and statistics is the results. While structure may vary somewhat, the research report usually includes an introductory section, methodology, results, and summary/conclusion. The results section reviews the outcomes when methodology is applied to data. Results may be inconclusive or nonsignificant (also sometimes referred to as negative results), significant/positive (matching predictions), significant/unpredicted (opposed to those predicted), mixed, or unexpected (not hypothesized).

125. B: When considering carrying out a health impact assessment (HIA), the initial action should be screening in order to identify projects that would benefit from an HIA. Screening is followed by scoping, which involves determining the health effects to assess. Then risks are assessed and benefits identified for those affected by the project and recommendations made regarding proposal changes in order to mitigate negative health effects. Finally, the results of the HIA are presented to those making decisions and evaluation is completed regarding the effect of the HIA on decisions.

126. D: The Framingham study in which a group of participants are monitored for a period of 20 years with a number of different variables assessed is categorized as a prospective study because the cause may have occurred, but the effect may not. For example, if a participant is obese and does not exercise, these risk factors may not have produced heart disease or diabetes, but these diseases still may occur at some future point.

127. D: Frieden's six components for effective public health program implementation include utilizing a limited number (rather than a large number) of high-priority evidence-based interventions. Other components include utilizing innovation for development of the evidence base, utilizing both partnerships and coalitions, obtaining the necessary resources and support, utilizing effective program management, and communicating accurate and timely information.

128. C: According to the 5 steps involved in the RE-AIM framework from translating research into intervention, the first step (R) refers to:

- R: reach the target population, aiming for the maximum number of participants
- E: efficacy, looking at both negative and positive factors
- A: adoption by target staff, organizations, and settings, including generating organizational/systemic support
- I: implementation consistency with a focus on fidelity
- M: maintenance of the program, focusing on sustainability

129. A: If a public health program to promote maternal and child health focuses on various factors that affect health, including interpersonal, individual, socioeconomic, institutional, and policy, this is an example of an ecological framework (EF). The ecosystems services (ES) framework focuses on the link between the individual/organization and the environment. The Natural Step (TNS) is a framework that focuses on leading an organization toward sustainability. The human-environmental systems (HES) focuses on investigation of the interaction between the individual/organization and the environment.

130. D: If a health education specialist is active in a national organization that aims to improve the health of all Americans by increasing access to care, the focus is on health equity. Health equity aims to ensure that all people have equal access to knowledge and resources, such as health care and adequate nutrition, in order to optimize their health. Health equity does not focus on health equality because that is unattainable because of factors such as genetic and environmental as well as individual choice.

131. C: If a software program has been installed on computers used in an organization in order to monitor who is using the network and the files that are accessed, this type of security tool is an intrusion detection system. This type of system is especially important if the network data include confidential information. An intrusion detection system generally requires a password or other identifying information (fingerprint, retinal scan) in order to access the system.

132. D: The least effective method of communicating an advocacy position to a member of Congress is the mailed letter because mailed materials must go through a bioterrorism screening process before they are passed on the legislator. Telephone calls, FAXs, and emails are all effective methods of communication. It is important to use key words during communications, especially electronic, because they are evaluated for statistical purposes so that the legislator knows which issues are generating the most interest.

133. D: Health Education evolved as a true profession in the 1970s, at which time criteria for credentialing of health educators was established. The Role Delineation Project was funded in 1978 and subsequently the criteria for entry-level health educators were outlined. The roles of health educators (entry and advanced level) have been further defined in the decades since the 1970s. The first CHES exam was given in 1990, and the CHES certification program was accredited in 2008 with the first MCHES exam for advanced practice released in 2011.

134. D: Dropbox is a technology option that allows people who are collaborating on a project to share, collaborate, and synchronize documents over the internet. Dropbox allows storage and sharing of documents, files, videos, and photos. Dropbox has both individual and business accounts with no charge for basic individual accounts. Business accounts allow unlimited storage and file recovery, remote wipe, and the ability to manage employee accounts. Dropbox business also allows the account holder to limit access to folders to specific users.

135. B: If the health education specialist sees a need in a program but does not have the financial resources to provide for the need, the best initial approach is to explore grant opportunities. Grants may be available from local organizations, businesses, national organizations, state programs, and federal programs. While it may be possible to transfer funds intended for another part of the program to provide for this need, this approach may result in unexpected problems, and fundraising takes a considerable investment in time and effort.

136. D: If the health education specialist is recruiting individuals for implementation of a program, an acceptable question to ask during the interview is, "Why do you want this position?" because this is a job-related question. The health education specialist can ask only if a person needs accommodations, but not about disabilities, and should not ask questions about race, gender, religion, national origin, marital status, or other personal matters. An individual may be questioned about fluency in English (the ability to read, write, and converse) but not about whether it is a first language.

137. B: If the health education specialist must implement a program that will provide educational services to a primarily English-speaking group, but a small subgroup in one community comprises Mexican immigrants with no or little English skills, the best approach is to provide materials in English and Spanish. While it may not always be possible to accommodate every non-English speaker, an effort should be made to do so when there is a subgroup speaking the same language.

138. A: If as part of program implementation, the electrical wiring must be modified in order to accommodate new technology needs, the most important criterion when selecting a person to do the work is licensure/certification. For legal safety reasons, a person working with electrical wiring should be a licensed electrician rather than a handyman with wiring experience. The health education specialist should always try to hire a professional because the licensure/certification/credential provides some assurance that the person has necessary education or skills.

139. C: If the health education specialist has facilitated a partnership between two organizations and wants to ensure that the partnership will be effective, the health education specialist should establish an evaluation plan. The plan should be completed as part of the preliminary preparation before the partnership is formalized and should include methods for recording and tracking data, reporting results, and evaluating progress toward goals and objectives, which should be agreed upon by the participating organizations.

140. D: When reviewing evidence to justify implementation of a program, the best source for systematic reviews is the Cochrane Library, which provides 7 different databases, including the *Cochrane Database of Systematic Reviews*. This database is updated continuously as new reports are available. Other databases that may be helpful are the *Database of Abstracts of Reviews of Effects* and the *Health Technology Assessment Database.*

141. B: If, when conducting a preliminary assessment of a community, the health education specialist drives through the community and observes the people (race, genders, dress, activities) and the places (boundaries, environment, buildings, housing), this type of assessment is referred to as a windshield survey. A windshield survey is a good method to use to get a general impression of the community because it is easy, fast, and inexpensive, but it should be followed by a more in-depth assessment.

142. A: If the health education specialist working in a community program to improve the health of mothers and babies finds that Chinese women in the community stay essentially bedridden for extended periods after giving birth and refuse to bathe or eat or drink cold foods, these practices are based on the health belief system referred to as humoral. The humoral health belief is concerned with balance between different forces, such as hot and cold. The Chinese women, then, avoid anything that may cause the body to lose heat, such as bathing or drinking cold liquids.

143. C: Population-based public health practice focuses on interventions at all levels, including those for the individual (family members or other at-risk groups with which the person is affiliated), the community (the entire population of a community or a subgroup within that community), and systems (laws, polices, and power structures). Population-based practice, a multilevel intervention program, attempts to take all of these different levels into consideration and to develop different interventions as necessary.

144. B: According to the attribution model of communication, an example of internal attribution is when an individual has lost 10 pounds and believes it is because she stayed on a diet and exercised. Internal attribution reflects the desire to see oneself in a positive light and to credit oneself for positive outcomes, such as weight loss. External attribution, on the other hand, refers to the belief that external events (such as the actions of another) influence outcomes.

145. C: If the health education specialist promotes alliances among a number of community agencies with similar interests, this is an example of coalition building. While each agency in a coalition maintains its self-interest, it also works cooperatively with other agencies to identify shared interests and solutions to problems as well as to prevent unnecessary overlapping of services. Coalitions are often temporary in nature and usually lack the formal obligations required of partnerships.

146. D: The purpose of social marketing is to influence attitudes, beliefs, and practices of a priority population with an aim to benefit that population by influencing their behavior. Social marketing is a critical factor in gaining cooperation with a priority population when implementing a program. Members of the population must recognize that a need exists in order to be open to the solution. Social marketing is similar to business marketing in that it includes the 4 Ps of product, price, place, and promotion.

147. A: Teaching individuals about nutritional food choices is an example of a cognitive intervention utilized in health teaching. Cognitive interventions involve provision of information and the acts of knowing, perceiving, and understanding. Affective interventions, on the other hand, are focused on feelings, attitudes, and values, such as helping individual to understand their fears or reassuring family members. Behavioral interventions focus on teaching specific skills, such as how to carry out a specific task.

148. D: The section of the research report that is likely to be most significant for readers is the summary/conclusion. In fact, this may be the only section that the reader actually reads, especially when conducting a review of the literature, because the summary/conclusion should contain the most important results derived from the research as well as suggestions for further research. Focusing on the summary/conclusion is a good method of eliminating research that is not applicable to a project.

149. C: When communicating with a visually impaired individual, the speaker should speak to the individual while approaching so that the individual is not startled. The speaker should use a normal tone of voice but should speak facing the person to aid in lip-reading. The speaker should describe activities and inform the person when the speaker is leaving the room. Adaptive materials, such as large print materials, may be needed, depending on the degree of visual impairment.

150. D: If the health education specialist is interested in applying for a grant to expand health services in a rural health program, the agency that may provide a grant is HRSA (Health Resources and Services Administration). HRSA provides grants to improve health services in a number of areas, including maternal and child health, HIV/AIDS, and rural health. HRSA is part of the US Department of Health and Human Services and aims to improve access to health care to those who are isolated geographically or are economically or medically disadvantaged.

151. A: When using Learning-Focused Advocacy Evaluation, the first step is to outline the purpose of the evaluation. The methodology may be influenced by the reason for the evaluation, and this should be clear at the outset. For example, if a grant requires specific information, then the evaluation must include that information. At this point, it is also important to determine the audience for the evaluation as this may influence the type of reporting that will be required.

152. B: If individuals at a clinic report that they believe HIV/AIDS rates have fallen, these are individual opinions and are not community-level indicators, which must focus on the community as a whole. Community-level indicators include area physicians who reported a 50% increase in prescriptions for Truvada for PrEP because Truvada markedly decreases risk of infection. Free clinics that reported an increase in requests for testing may indicate more awareness, and the public health department's report of a 40% decrease in HIV/AIDS infections shows that goals are being met.

153. C: The URL domain extension that the health education specialist should advise individuals is the least valid when searching for information about health is .com, which is the most commonly used generic extension for individuals and businesses, including email and social media.

Organizations typically use .org as the URL extension, but care must be used when determining the validity of the organization. The URL extension .edu is used by education institutions and sometimes by their students, while .gov, the most reliable, is used by government agencies and .mil by the military.

154. D: If the health education specialist is assessing a priority population's need for health-related information and is reviewing economic indicators, such as unemployment rates, the best resource is the US Census Bureau. Unemployment rates are available as part of labor force statistics. The US Census Bureau reports on a wide range of economic indicators that may provide information about social determinants of health, such as homeownership and rental vacancy rates, new residential construction, and retail trade.

155. A: If, when advocating for change in the delivery of care to older adults, the health education specialist finds that one insurance representative routinely questions the right of the health education specialist to address the issue and claims that no real problems exist, the tactic that the insurance representative is using is discounting. Discrediting involves questioning the advocate's motives. Dulcifying refers to offers of jobs, payments, or other benefits in order to pacify an advocate. Deflecting is changing the focus or passing the issue on to someone with no power to resolve it.

156. D: If an individual is able to slowly read directions out loud but, when questioned, the person clearly does not understand the meaning enough to carry out the directions, the individual would be classified as having functional illiteracy because the person lacks the basic skills in reading, writing, and understanding that are needed to function well in society. It is important when working with individuals who lack literacy to remember that literacy does not necessarily equate to intelligence. Some people lack the opportunity to learn, and others have learning disabilities that interfere with learning.

157. B: A company newsletter would be classified as an organizational channel of communication. Other activities in the organizational channel of communication include meetings and conferences, campaigns in the workplace (such as no-smoking or weight reduction), in-house radio/video productions, or add-on messages (such as a memo attached to a paystub). While organizational channels may be trusted and influential and can easily reach the target population, there may be organizational limitations and efforts can be time consuming.

158. C: If a local television station has agreed to run public service ads for an educational program the health education specialist is implementing in the community, the first question the health education specialist should ask is: "What hours and how frequently will the ads run?" Media outlets generally place PSAs in unsold time slots and these are rarely available during prime time, so the ads may run in the middle of the night. Additionally, a good ad can be costly to produce, so a free placement is not the same as a free ad.

159. D: An individual who is paid to actively seek to influence a senator's vote on a public health issue by representing an organization and providing information and statistics is a lobbyist, who must comply with the Lobbying Disclosure Act. An advocate, on the other hand, usually makes a less direct appeal in order to increase awareness of issues. The terms, however, are not mutually exclusive, as an advocate may also be a lobbyist or may support lobbying efforts. Lobbyists are often paid while advocates generally are not.

160. B: The WK Kellogg Foundation (wkkf.org) is a health philanthropic agency, but it does not provide information about advocacy evaluation. The Innovation Network (innont.org) is a clearinghouse for evaluation, research, and consulting, and provides numerous advocacy evaluation resources and tools. This source has the most extensive resources to aid in advocacy evaluation, including a logic model builder and an evaluation plan builder that utilizes data from the model builder to create evaluation questions. The California Endowment (calendow.org) also contains some information about advocacy and evaluation as does the Evaluation Exchange (hfrp.org).

161. A: The level of system change that is involved when the health education specialist attempts to change the basic mindset of beliefs or individuals regarding how a system works is the paradigm. A paradigm shift can be difficult to bring about because of entrenched belief systems and the need to view matters from a different perspective. A system for change may attempt to shift the paradigm or may, in fact, reinforce the paradigm, depending on the focus of change.

162. B: If a free health clinic for Mexican migrant farm workers is located near migrant housing and operates from Monday to Friday from 8 AM to 5 PM but attendance has been poor, the most likely reason for the poor use of the facility is the hours of business. Most farm workers work from dawn to dusk, so services to this population need to be provided with flexible hours, such as in the evening or very early in the morning.

163. A: When determining the feasibility of implementing recommendations for changes based on a health impact assessment (HIA), multiple factors must be considered. These factors can include the cost of implementing the recommendations and the funds available, the resources needed to implement change (materials, staff, and equipment), the policies in place that may impact implementation, the political situation and support or lack of support, the time needed to carry out the changes, and the general context.

164. A: Pilot studies should be conducted in settings similar to those where the intervention will be used. This is critical if the data derived from the pilot study is to be of value as the conclusions may not be generalizable if the setting is substantially different. For example, if an educational program is to be available to a number of community organizations, then one small organization may be selected for the pilot. The participants should, if possible, be representative of the priority population.

165. B: According to the systems approach to organizational change (Rowitz), the first stage is to clarify values, such as through conducting a culture audit. The next stage is to construct or revise the mission and vision statements to reflect the desired changes and then to identify goals and objectives. At this point, the action plan can be developed and implemented, followed by evaluation of the program to determine if it is successful or requires modification.

It's Your Moment, Let's Celebrate It!

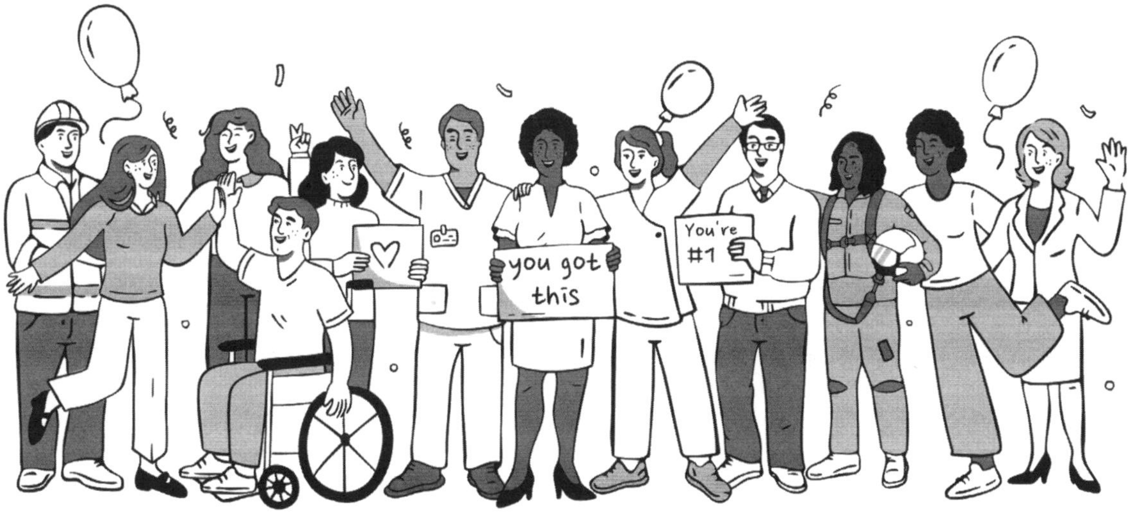

Share your story @mometrixtestpreparation